Organisational Capacity Building in Health Systems

T0227933

Capacity building focuses on understanding the obstacles that prevent organisations from realising their goals, while promoting those features that help them to achieve measurable and sustainable results. It is vital for improving the delivery of health care in both developed and developing countries. Organisations are important structural building blocks of health systems because they provide platforms for delivery of curative and preventive health services, and facilitate health workforce financing and functions.

Organisational capacity building involves more than training and equipment and this book discusses management capacity to realign systems, structures and roles strategically to optimise organisational performance in health care. Examining the topic in a practical and comprehensive way, *Organisational Capacity Building in Health Systems* is divided into five parts, looking at:

- what health organisations are and do;
- management and leadership in health organisations;
- how to build capacity in health systems;
- building capacity in a range of health system contexts;
- dealing with challenges in building capacity and evaluating work.

Examining how to effectively design, implement and evaluate organisational capacity building initiatives, this book is ideal for public health, health promotion and health management researchers, students and practitioners.

Niyi Awofeso is Professor in the School of Population Health, University of Western Australia, and Conjoint Professor in the School of Public Health and Community Medicine, University of New South Wales.

Routledge studies in public health

Organisational Capacity Building in Health Systems

Niyi Awofeso

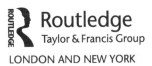

Routledge
Taylor & Francis Group

LONDON AND NEW YORK

First published 2013
by Routledge

2 Park Square, Milton Park, Abingdon, Oxon OX14 4RN
711 Third Avenue, New York, NY 10017, USA

Routledge is an imprint of the Taylor & Francis Group, an informa business

First issued in paperback 2017

British Library Cataloguing in Publication Data
A catalogue record for this book is available from the British Library

Library of Congress Cataloging in Publication Data
Awofeso, Niyi.
Organisational capacity building in health systems / Niyi Awofeso.
  p. cm. – (Routledge studies in public health)
  Includes bibliographical references.
  I. Title. II. Series: Routledge studies in public health.
  [DNLM: 1. Delivery of Health Care–organization &
  administration. 2. Capacity Building. 3. Health Services
  Administration. W 84.1]
  LC classification not assigned
  362.1–dc23   2012008702
ISBN: 978-0-415-52179-6 (hbk)
ISBN: 978-1-138-11685-6 (pbk)

Typeset in Baskerville
by Wearset Ltd, Boldon, Tyne and Wear

To Emeritus Professor Pieter Degeling – my teacher, mentor, guardian and friend

Contents

Figures

Tables

Prologue

By the end of their two-year placement, Indonesia's Yayasan Peduli Munti Gunung (YPMG) foundation had established strong management structures, and secured funding for educational, medical and housing projects. And while Dave and Christine Cloughley are now enjoying their retirement in the traditional Aussie way – by touring the country in a caravan – they continue to advise and support YPMG from afar. Says Dave: 'Volunteering is a great way to start retirement; knowing we have made a contribution to capacity building in a developing country and that we have been able to make a difference to people's lives.'

Weekend Australian Magazine, 5 October 2011

'Capacity building' is a conceptual approach to organisational development that focuses on understanding and surmounting the obstacles that encumber organisations from realising their development goals while enhancing the abilities that allow them to achieve measurable and sustainable results. The field of organisational capacity building has its origins in the realms of practice, not in an academic discipline. Like Dave and Christine Cloughley in the quote above, anyone able to contribute substantially to fostering efficient organisational structures, skilled human resources in the right mix and distribution, and sustainable financing of organisations, is an organisational capacity builder. Capacity building is very relevant to ongoing efforts to reform health systems globally. The call for health organisations to build capacity has become more strident in the past several decades as more money and global interest are devoted to health care provision, even in developing nations. The more technical aspects of organisational capacity building – such as training and tools/equipment – are relatively easy to address. In contrast, structures, systems and roles require sharper definition and addressing these aspects of organisational capacity building remain problematic.

This book explores the topic of capacity building from five thematic perspectives: theories, typologies and functions of organisations (Chapters 1–4), management practices which may facilitate or encumber capacity building efforts (Chapters 5–6), conceptual framework and intervention points (Chapters 7–8), context-specific capacity building policies, programmes and practices (Chapters 9–18) and evaluation methods for capacity building (Chapters 19–20). The book explores dated and contemporary concepts, as well as the science and art, of capacity building. Also discussed are challenges faced in current capacity building efforts, and practical recommendations to improve and advance disciplinary and interdisciplinary capacity initiatives. This book is recommended for public health students, managers of civil society organisations and managers in health organisations who have an interest, or stake, in capacity building.

Part I

Theories, typology and functions of organisations

1 Evolution of capacity building concept in health systems

While working as a volunteer infectious diseases physician at Kyrgyzstan's prisons in 2007, I developed an epiphany on why the concept of 'capacity building' in health systems is so challenging, and yet so important. While Kyrgyzstan struggled to develop a new political framework following the implosion of the former Soviet Union, it had virtually lost control of the health and security management of its 16,000 prisoners. Criminal leaders transformed large sections of prisoners into armies in reserve. Violence, transmission of multi-drug resistant tuberculosis infection among prisoners and eventually from prisoners to their relatives and close contacts in the general community, were common. The tuberculosis control situation was so deplorable that two leading international non-governmental health movements – International Committee of the Red Cross and Doctors Without Borders – took over responsibility for prevention and treatment of tuberculosis and other public health problems in prison settings.

I realised that in order to restore normalcy to Kyrgyzstan government's management of prison health services, it is important to develop indigenous capacity – i.e. enhance the capability of the people and government of Kyrgyzstan to undertake stated objectives – for effective management of prisons at institutional, human rights, judicial and public health perspectives. Institutional capacity building in Kyrgyzstan prisons' context entails reforms of penal financing, infrastructure, personnel, security, corruption and dissolution of the 'obshchak' system of prison gang-led, violence-prone, prison management. At the human rights level, most incidents of violence and abuse inflicted by police and prison staff on inmates are apparently condoned by custodial authorities, and this has created a vicious cycle of payback violent attacks by inmates on other inmates and occasionally on custodial workers, including nurses and doctors. Training, employment and retention of health workers of the right mix, as well as equitable distribution of health workers and facilities within the prison system require carefully coordinated interdisciplinary capacity building efforts. Justice reforms include restoring the observance of the rule of law, especially by crime investigators, who are widely perceived as torturing crime suspects in order to obtain evidence. At the prisoner health care level, the fragile building blocks of health care delivery to prisoners – quality workforce, drugs and equipment, information technology, governance – crumbled with the demise of the former Soviet Union, and have been neglected since the late 1980s.[1]

Although the decision by international non-governmental health-related organisations to address the worsening tuberculosis situation in Kyrgyzstan's prisons was commendable and urgently required by prison inmates and staff at risk of contracting or dying from tuberculosis,[2] it addressed only a minor facet of the organisational capacity building processes required for transforming Kyrgyzstan's prison system. It would have been impractical for health-focussed civil society groups to address non-health components of Kyrgyzstan's prison capacity building components, but it is vitally important for all stakeholders to work in unison towards this goal, as piecemeal approaches to capacity building have, in general, unsatisfactory track records. Capacity development is a fundamental part of the mandates of many international organisations. Much of their activities aim to strengthen national capacities through training, technical advice, exchange of experiences, research and policy advice. Yet there is considerable dissatisfaction within the international community regarding the impact of many such interventions. Within the health sector, training-centred activities of international aid agencies have usually strengthened the skills of individuals, but have not always succeeded in improving the effectiveness of the ministries and other organisations where those individuals are working.[3]

For example, Haiti had about 5,000 non-governmental organisations working on various projects prior to the devastating January 2010 earthquake. Following the earthquake, millions of dollars were donated for emergency relief, and the number of civil society groups in Haiti increased to over 7,000. Yet, two years following the earthquake, there is estimated to be only one toilet for every 200 people in the Port au Prince metropolitan area. Water shortage is the norm. Electricity supply is epileptic. Poverty is endemic. Social services such as education and security are equally grossly inadequate or of substandard quality. In Africa, General Siad Barre was ousted as Somali president in 1991. While the lack of an existing political order and institutions of government (including administrative structures at the local, state and national levels) allowed authority to remain in the hands of competing warlords and clans, it became very difficult to meet the essential preconditions for effective post-conflict reconstruction and provision of health services in Somalia. Currently, Somalia is a failed state in the grip of severe famine, and its life expectancy at birth is estimated at 49 years. It has the highest rank for terrorism risk in the 2011 Maplecroft terrorism index. One lesson from the poor outcomes in relation to Haiti's and Somalia's reconstruction is that when a government is grossly ineffective, it needs to be reformed from bottom-up before reconstruction programmes can be successful. While short-term gains may be achieved within the health systems of failed states through vertical programmes, such as measles immunisation delivery, such vertical programmes are generally unsustainable and may further weaken vulnerable health systems. As Bill Gates perhaps belatedly realised following the resurgence of polio in Tajikistan and other Asian countries where it had been declared eradicated, and following two decades and $8.3 billion dollars to eradicate the disease:

> Is humanity better served by waging wars on individual diseases, like polio? Or is it better to pursue a broader set of health goals simultaneously – improving hygiene, expanding immunizations, providing clean drinking water – that don't eliminate any one disease, but might improve the overall health of people in developing countries? The new plan integrates both approaches. It's an acknowledgment, bred by last summer's outbreak, that disease-specific wars can succeed only if they also strengthen the overall health system in poor countries.[4]

From around the 1960s, 'nation building' was promoted by international agencies as a way to ensure that newly independent nations were able to develop appropriate social, legal, economic, health, judicial and political structures to facilitate long-term development. The conventional idea of nation building has always revolved around that of an externally driven top-down structure meant for the express purpose of state and administrative reconstruction. Especially in nations emerging from conflict or natural disasters, such nation building approaches tend to be of a 'practical' nature, focussing on infrastructural reconstruction, humanitarian assistance in terms of food and medical supplies, construction of roads, schools, health care provision, and expansion of water and sewage treatment facilities. Nation building in this context was thus viewed as a rehabilitation campaign which is expected to 'provide the physical and organisational infrastructure populations need to re-establish normal lives'.[5]

For more stable, but underdeveloped, nations, the United Nations Development Programme (UNDP) promoted the concept of 'Institution Building' in the 1970s, as a platform for facilitating long-term prosperity, security and health outcomes. Keohane defines institutions as the 'persistent and connected set of rules that prescribe behavioural roles, constrain activities, and shape expectations'.[6] While specific institutions can be defined in the first instance in terms of rules, it should be recognised that their effects are also embedded in 'practices', i.e. manner of individual and administrative behaviour towards citizens and other agencies of government within the state. It became apparent to the UNDP in the 1980s and 1990s that it is possible that the prevailing institutional architecture could be the source of continued misunderstanding among stakeholders, in the same way that societal and cultural differences are. This made the top-down UNDP approach to development difficult to justify. The following quote, from East Timorese independence leader Xanana Gusmao, highlights the inherent contradictions of the institution building approach in delivering community participation in newly independent East Timor:

> We are not interested in a legacy of cars and laws, nor are we interested in a legacy of development plans for Timorese … We are not interested in inheriting an economic rationale which leaves out the social and political complexity of East Timorese reality. Nor do we wish to inherit the heavy decision-making and project implementation mechanisms in which the role of the East Timorese is to give their consent as observers rather than the active players we should start to be.[7]

The concept of 'capacity building' (otherwise stated as 'capacity development') replaced 'institution building' in the lexicon of international development organisations from the mid-1990s onwards. 'Capacity building' implies a focus on the existing capacities of governments and how these capacities can become strengthened on all levels – the individual, the organisational and the institutional, as well as the broader system context. Governments, donor agencies and international organisations involved in development are increasingly putting an emphasis on capacities as key to sustainable development. Capacity building entails the activities and structures that leverage existing resources in pursuit of some common objective(s), and which are sustainable over the long term. The process of capacity building is expected to improve the ability of a person, group, organisation or system to meet identified objectives or to perform better.

In the health sector, the concept of capacity building has gained increasing currency over the past decade. The United States Agency for International Development (USAID) capacity building for health framework focuses on the management, organisational and business planning competencies essential to sustainable health care organisations. It includes six core organisational competencies. *Technical expertise*: does the organisation have the technical capacity to carry out its mandate? This includes the ability to access tools and methodologies and a technically qualified workforce. *Resource mobilisation*: does the organisation have a business model that allows it to mobilise resources and be financially viable? *Technical assistance and training*: do local staff and consultants have basic skills in consulting and training to provide effective technical assistance and training? *Management systems*: does the organisation have the necessary management systems in areas such as financial management, procurement, human resources and administration to function effectively? *Organisational development*: does the organisation have the capacity to plan and manage its activities? This includes the ability to develop strategic and operational plans, provide effective leadership and management, build an effective team and create a structure with clear roles and responsibilities. Finally, *Governance*: is there a governance system that provides the necessary checks and balances?[8]

In a 2001 document published by the New South Wales (Australia) Health Department (NSWHEALTH), capacity building was defined as: 'An approach to the development of sustainable skills, organisational structures, resources and commitment to health improvement in health and other sectors, to prolong and multiply health gains many times over.' They adopted the capacity building framework shown in Figure 1.1.

The perspective on capacity building adopted in this book is a hybrid of the USAID and NSWHEALTH frameworks. From health research strengthening[10] to enhancing collaborative and productive partnerships between civil society groups,[11] capacity building is increasingly being promoted as a mainstream concept in health systems strengthening. However, to date, emphasis on capacity building in health professional education remains inadequate in depth and scope. The chapters in this book seek to contribute to raising awareness of the role of capacity building in health systems strengthening in general and in the successful management of health programmes and services in particular. Obstacles to widespread adoption of capacity building concepts in health systems are discussed, and methods for assessing the impact of capacity building initiatives are highlighted. The building blocks and theoretical frameworks of capacity building are explored, in order to make precepts easier to adapt to readers' contexts.

The tremendous success of the post-1986 global Guinea worm eradication programme illustrates the practical application of the capacity building concept in health systems development. Public health efforts to control Guinea worm (*Dracunculus medinensis*) date back to 1980 when the

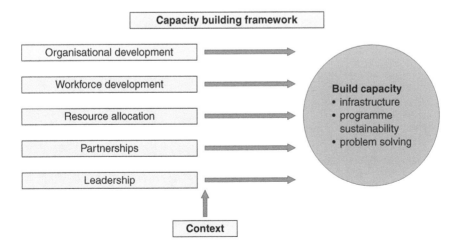

Figure 1.1 Capacity building framework (adapted from reference 9).

World Health Organization (WHO) instituted the Decade of Safe Water and Sanitation. Guinea worm was targeted for control during the 1980s. Guinea worm is a disease known since antiquity. Its presence was confirmed by histological examination of Egyptian mummies from the early part of the first millennium BC.[12] Guinea worm affects primarily the rural populations because of their dependency on open wells, ponds and rivers for drinking water. Traditionally, these populations have been neglected economically, socially and health-wise. Because of the disease, women were unable to care normally for themselves, their children or their households, or do other work that would add income to the family. Children suffering from the disease miss school, and the effects of their repeated absences show up negatively in their academic performance. The life cycle of Guinea worm makes rural populations particularly prone to infection (Figures 1.2 and 1.3).

Following a 1984 visit to Pakistan by former American President Jimmy Carter where only two cases of Guinea worm had been reported by national health authorities but the local health worker informed him that he had treated about 1,200 cases,[13] Carter revitalised the WHO Guinea worm eradication initiative, and made Guinea worm eradication a core programme of the Carter Center, a non-governmental organisation he founded in 1982. His first major breakthrough was endorsement, in 1986, of Pakistan's President and Vice President's initiative for a county-wide Guinea worm eradication programme, assisted by the Carter Center's Global 2000. At the time, there were about 3.5 million annual cases of the disease in 21 countries in Africa and Asia. Capacity building initiatives for Guinea worm eradication included the following:[14,15,16]

- Demonstration of effective transformational leadership by Jimmy Carter, in part by drawing on his substantial political capital as former President of the United States to bring Guinea worm eradication to the forefront of international disease control efforts. In 1989, WHO's forty-second

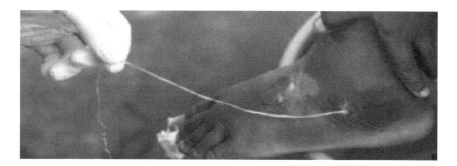

Figure 1.2 Adult Guinea worm being taken out of a patient's leg (picture credit: The Carter Foundation).

World Health Assembly declared the goal of eliminating Guinea worm as a public health problem from the world during the 1990s and endorsed a strategy for realising this goal. It was only the third time in its history that the WHO had slated a disease for eradication.

- The Carter Center's strong technical, fundraising, prevention, treatment and surveillance partnerships for Guinea worm control with reputable organisations, such as the Centers for Disease Control and Prevention (CDC), the WHO, UNICEF and the Bill and Melinda Gates Foundation. These international partnerships were further amplified by national and community partnerships encouraged by the Carter Center to stimulate intersectoral collaboration and community participation in health.
- Jimmy Carter worked with stakeholders at international, national and community levels to ensure that adequate financial and technical resources were made available for Guinea worm eradication efforts. For example, in 1989, UNDP donated US$1 million, UNICEF donated US$1.55 million and US$9.6 million was raised at an international Guinea worm conference in Nigeria, including US$1 million from the government of Nigeria for its own Guinea worm eradication programme.

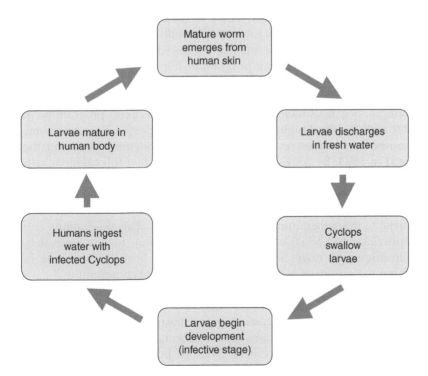

Figure 1.3 Life cycle of *Dracunculus medinensis.*

- Workforce development was tailored to the unique features of the disease. Unlike smallpox or syphilis, the key to eradication lies not in vaccines or drugs, but in community education and action. Guinea worm can be eradicated only through an intensive community effort. The people at risk have the primary responsibility for taking the personal and community actions that have proved effective. For example, in Togo, the Guinea worm eradication goals were set for 50 Carter Center and CDC volunteers who were working on the project from January 1992. They were expected to have achieved the following milestones by December 1996: (i) train and mobilise at least 9,100 nationals (health workers, teachers, members of village development committees) operating in villages where Guinea worm is endemic to participate actively in the national effort to eliminate the disease; (ii) reduce to 0 per cent the incidence of Guinea worm in the villages where the volunteers were working. These two goals were achieved prior to the target date.
- Organisational development activities were undertaken at international, national and community levels to facilitate the Guinea worm eradication effort. At international level, the Carter Center created the Guinea worm eradication department, headed by Professor Donald Hopkins, Vice President of Carter Center Health programmes, and five other technical staff. These technical staff continue to liaise with national governments to develop public–private partnerships for Guinea worm eradication efforts.[17] The CDC and WHO provide further technical support for programme implementation. At national levels, 'vertical' Guinea worm eradication programmes were encouraged, supported with dedicated staff and funding. Uganda, for example, began its national Guinea worm eradication programme in 1991 with the third-highest number of cases reported by any endemic country, and ranked as the second-highest endemic country in the world in 1993. By 2004, Uganda celebrated its first full calendar year with no indigenous cases of the disease. Strong organisational development, support of the 'vertical' eradication programme and dedicated leadership by government officials and external partners were crucial to this programme's remarkable success. This programme cost approximately US$5.6 million, a small investment for a disease that, following worm extraction, takes six weeks to heal thus resulting in substantial productivity losses particularly in rural communities.[18]

Largely as a result of organisational capacity building efforts for Guinea worm control, the number of cases dropped drastically from 3.5 million in 21 countries in 1986 to 1,797 cases in four African countries – Sudan, Mali, Ethiopia and Ghana – by December 2010. In July 2011, Ghana formally eradicated Guinea worm after a 23-year campaign. Guinea worm disease remains endemic in newly independent South Sudan and in pockets of Mali and Ethiopia. Chad also recently experienced an isolated outbreak. A total of 804 cases were reported in those countries as at 30 August 2011.[17]

The sustainability of the Guinea worm eradication capacity building programme is attested to by the rarity of Guinea worm resurgence in areas where it has been declared eradicated. This is largely due to the bottom-up capacity building approach whereby local communities are motivated to act and prevent contamination of drinking water by Guinea worm larvae. Guinea worm is likely to be the second human infectious disease to be eradicated. The capacity building approach which has barely literate but highly motivated volunteer village workers as its frontline staff has proved a successful and revolutionary approach to public health management in poor communities. The programme has enhanced the credibility of international health organisations, national health systems and local health workers, and exemplifies the potential of expert adoption of organisational capacity building approaches in health systems development.

References

1 International Crisis Group. Kyrgyzstan prison system nightmare. Asia Report No. 118, 16 August 2006. Available from: www.crisisgroup.org/~/media/Files/asia/central-asia/kyrgyzstan/118_kyrgyzstans_prison_system_nightmare.pdf (accessed 21 September 2011).

2 Mokrousov, I., Valcheva, V., Sovhozova, N., Aldashev, A., Rastogi, N., Isakova, J. Penitentiary population of Mycobacterium tuberculosis in Kyrgyzstan: exceptionally high prevalence of the Beijing genotype and its Russia-specific subtype. *Infection, Genetics and Evolution*, 2009; 9: 1400–1405.

3 Ulleberg, I. *The Role and Impact of NGOs in Capacity Development: From Replacing the State to Reinvigorating Education.* Paris: International Institute for Educational Planning, 2009.

4 Guth, R.A. Gates rethinks his war on polio. *Wall Street Journal* (Health Industry section), 23 April 2010.

5 Serafino, N.M. Peacekeeping and related stability operations: issues of US military involvement, CRS Issue Brief for Congress, IB94040, 27 March 2006, pp. 1–15.

6 Keohane, R. International institutions: two research programs. *International Studies Quarterly*, 1988; 32: 379–396.

7 Beauvais, J.C. Benevolent despotism: a critique of UN state building in East Timor. *International Law and Politics*, 2001; 33: 1101–1178.

8 United States Agency for International Development. *Health Systems 20.20.* Washington DC: USAID, 2009. Available from: www.healthsystems2020.org/ (accessed 21 September 2011).

9 New South Wales Health Department. *A Framework for Building Capacity to Improve Health.* Sydney: NSWHEALTH, 2001.

10 Mahmood, S., Hort, K., Ahmed, S., Salam, M., Cravioto, A. Strategies for capacity building for health research in Bangladesh: role of core funding and a common monitoring and evaluation framework. *Health Research Policy and Systems*, 2011; 9: 31.

11 Alexander, J.A., Christianson, J.B., Hearld, L.R., Hurley, R., Scanlon, D.P. Challenges of capacity building in multi-sector community health alliances. *Health Education and Behaviour*, 2010; 37: 645–664.

12 Burdick, W.P., Morahan, P.S., Norcini, J.J. Capacity building in medical education and health outcomes in developing countries: the missing link. *Education for Health*, 2007; 65, Epub 20 November 2007.

13 Adamson, P.B. Dracontiasis in antiquity. *Medical History*, 1988; 32: 204–209.

14 Select Committee on Hunger. *United States House of Representatives Eradication of Guinea Worm Disease*. Washington, DC: US Government Printing Office, 1987, p. 5.

15 Yolahem, D., Benjamin, J.G., Olson, P. *Programming Guide for Guinea Worm Eradication*. US Agency for International Development under WASH Task No. 091. Washington DC: USAID, 1990.

16 Barry, M. The tail end of Guinea worm: global eradication without a drug or a vaccine. *New England Journal of Medicine*, 2007; 356: 2561–2564.

17 Carter Center. *Countdown to Zero: Guinea Worm Disease Eradication*. Atlanta: Carter Center, 2011. Available from: www.cartercenter.org/health/guinea_worm/mini_site/index.html (accessed 24 September 2011).

18 Rwakimari, J.B., Hopkins, D.R., Ruiz-Tiben, E. Uganda's successful Guinea worm eradication programme. *American Journal of Tropical Medicine and Hygiene*, 2006; 75: 3–8.

2 Health systems

From microscope to telescope: (re)defining 'health'

At the official launch of the Research Network on Health Systems and Infection in May 2011, co-founder Greg Reilly stated that: 'in recent years there has been a growing momentum towards looking beyond the biological causes of infection towards a better understanding of those systematic mechanisms that contribute to, or prevent, infection and disease'.[1] Understanding the structure and function of health systems are prerequisites for acquiring adequate knowledge of appropriate health protection and disease prevention interventions. However, it is important to first clarify what 'health' means. Health is defined in the World Health Organization (WHO) constitution of 1948 as: 'A state of complete physical, social and mental well-being, and not merely the absence of disease or infirmity.'[2] This definition has not been amended since. WHO's definition widened the domain of health from the physical to the social and mental realms, and it made explicit that disease and infirmity, when isolated from subjective experience, are inadequate to qualify health. At the conceptual level, when conflicts between health needs and available health resources are of paramount concern, this definition becomes problematic. According to Saracci:

> a state of complete physical, mental, and social wellbeing corresponds much more closely to happiness than to health. These two words designate distinct life experiences. Sigmund Freud, an appropriate reference in psychological matters, saw it clearly when, after stopping smoking cigars for health reasons, he wrote: 'I learned that health was to be had at a certain cost.... Thus I am now better than I was, but not happier.'[3]

However, Saracci's definition – 'Health is a condition of well-being free of disease or infirmity and a basic and universal human right' – has not fared better. For instance, should society regard the one billion people currently living with a disability as unhealthy, or can disabled people who are otherwise joyful and well adjusted to their disability be described as healthy? It appears that, in relation to definition of health, Rufus Miles' aphorism – 'Where you stand depends on where you sit'[4] – applies. Health system managers are more likely to constrain the definitional scope of health in formulating health spending priorities, while consumers are more likely to base their perspective of health on the WHO definition. Were the goals set in 1948 too ambitious? Is health a construct that can be defined and measured? Is health, like beauty, in the eye of the beholder?

To answer these questions, a brief overview of the historical evolution of health is appropriate. Although concern with health and disease have been major preoccupations of humans since antiquity, the use of the word 'health' to describe human 'well-being' is relatively recent. The word 'health' was derived from the old English word 'hoelth', which meant a state of being sound, and was generally used to infer a soundness of the body.[5] Prior to the period of the somewhat enigmatic physician known as Hippocrates (*c.*460–377 BC), health was perceived as a divine gift. Hippocrates was credited with pioneering the move away from divine notions of health, and using observation as a basis for acquiring health knowledge. He was credited with encouraging a focus on environmental sanitation, personal hygiene and, in particular, balanced diets – 'let food be thy medicine; and let thy medicine be food'. He theorised that what we currently regard as 'health' might be defined as the extent of a delicate balance of four fluids: blood, yellow bile, black bile and phlegm. Ill health, he believed, resulted from an imbalance of these fluids.

Nevertheless, a divine view of health persists to this era. For example, Islam's Prophet Mohammed seemingly fatalistic view of health, sickness and death – followed by a high proportion of practising Muslims – may be inferred from the following verse in the Holy Koran; 'The Lord of the worlds; it is He who heals me when I am sick, and He who would cause me to die and live again' (Koran 26: 80). Health belief systems also influence perspectives on the meaning of health. For instance, Becker's Health Belief Model[6] might be used to explain differences in how the concept of health is perceived by individuals and groups – particularly in non-religious contexts – and how such perceptual differences influence response to ill health. Australian Aboriginal people generally define health thus 'Health does not just mean the physical well-being of the individual but refers to the social, emotional, spiritual and cultural well-being of the whole community. This is a whole of life view and includes the cyclical concept of life-death-life'[7] (see Figure 2.1).

Health is being increasingly considered less as an abstract state and more as a means to an end which can be expressed in functional terms as a resource which permits people to lead an individually, socially and economically productive life. Health is framed as a resource for everyday life, not the object of living. A comprehensive understanding of health implies that all systems and structures which govern social, political, religious, occupational

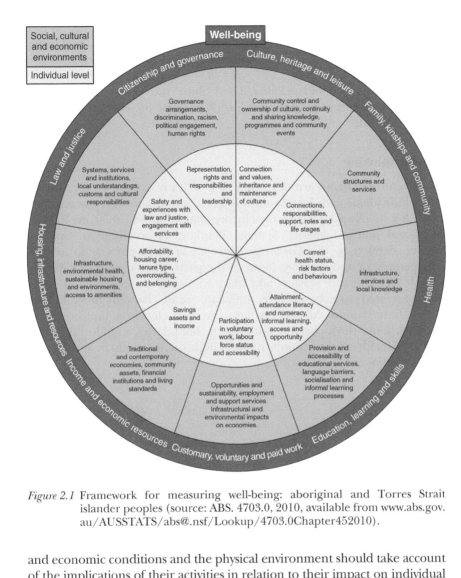

Figure 2.1 Framework for measuring well-being: aboriginal and Torres Strait islander peoples (source: ABS. 4703.0, 2010, available from www.abs.gov. au/AUSSTATS/abs@.nsf/Lookup/4703.0Chapter452010).

and economic conditions and the physical environment should take account of the implications of their activities in relation to their impact on individual and collective health and well-being. These variables may positively or negatively impact on individual and community health status, and are commonly referred to as Determinants of Health (Figure 2. 2).

In the author's view, a good definition of health for the twenty-first century should address five core facets: *negative*, i.e. as the absence of illness; *functional*, i.e. as ability to cope with everyday activities and life's stresses, as well as presence of joy when all is not well; *positive*, as fitness and well-being; *rights*, as opposed to charity; *dynamic*, as in variations throughout the life-course. Such a definition might read as:

Health is a dynamic state of physical, social and psychological well-being and not merely the absence of disease. Its basic provision is a human right, and it constitutes a vital resource both for optimal living and for coping with adverse events throughout the life-course.

The definitions and perspectives stated above introduce valuable additional concepts that may be used to enrich or revise the current WHO definition of health.

Systems thinking

Health and well-being are the result of a series of complex processes in which individuals and communities interact with others and the environment. A systems approach ensures incorporation of individual, ecological, social and political factors. Systems Thinking is premised on Systems Theory, defined by the *Cambridge Dictionary of Philosophy* (2002) as 'the arrangement of and relations between the parts which connect them into a whole'. Health care services take place within sub-systems such as acute care, extended care, home care, ambulatory care. Patients move in and out of these systems. All systems have common elements: input, output, feedback loop, throughput, environment, boundaries, equilibrium, constraints. Health administrators require high quality skills in integrating health systems components.

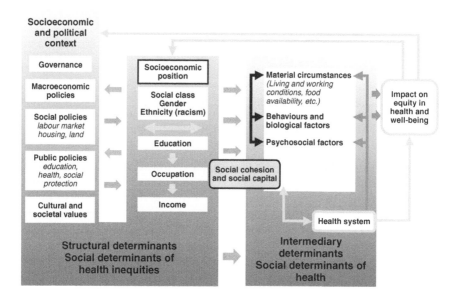

Figure 2.2 Conceptual framework for social determinants of health (adapted from WHO Social Determinants of Health Report, 2011).

Systems thinking is a process of estimating or inferring how local policies, actions or changes influence the state of the neighbouring and/or related policies or actions. It is an approach to problem solving, viewing 'problems' as parts of an overall system, rather than reacting to present outcomes or events and potentially contributing to further development of the undesired issue or problem. Systems thinking is a framework that is based on the belief that the component parts of a system can best be understood in the context of relationships with each other and with other systems, rather than in isolation. Systems thinking applies systems principles to aid a decision maker with problems of identifying, reconstructing, optimising and controlling a system, while taking into account multiple objectives, constraints and resources.[7]

Core components of Systems thinking are: (a) systems knowledge – involves trans-disciplinary understanding of 'causal', 'risk' or 'determinant' factors related to a given issue; (b) systems networks – understanding how these various facets are linked; and (c) systems methods – determining the most efficient and practical ways to facilitate collaborations between stakeholders, and utilise linkages to achieve sustainable outcomes. The context, circumstances and environment of a system play an important role in systems thinking. When systems get more complex due to more parts, actors, interactions and communication, the origin of problems gets harder to identify. Such complex 'social systems' are common in the health sector. For example, Indigenous Australians suffer disproportionately from cardiovascular diseases such as cardiomyopathy, diabetes and hypertension.[8] Addressing such complex health problems by focussing on individual facets is unlikely to be productive, given that it is the interactions and synergisms between the various factors which contribute to the high rates of vascular disease among Indigenous Australians. Application of Systems Thinking principles facilitates better understanding of the issues and suggests critical intervention points (Figure 2.3).

In relation to a major risky behaviour among Indigenous Australian youth – tobacco smoking – which, at 55 per cent, is three times the national average smoking prevalence,[9] a systems thinking approach helps to integrate intervention mechanisms (Figure 2.4).

Systems thinking is not only applicable to 'public health' sectors of the health system. In clinical settings, patient safety may be optimised with application of systems thinking orientation. In the United Kingdom, it is estimated that 10 per cent of hospital patients experience some form of clinical error and, annually, there could be as many as 850,000 of these events, costing the health service over £2 billion in additional care.[10] Triggers and opportunities for error located within the organisation can align and combine to enable human error and patient harm. The British National Patient Safety Agency lists systems thinking, framed as a fabric of cultural change – 'safety culture' – as the first of 'seven steps to patient safety'.[11] Common contributory 'systems' factors for patient safety are depicted in the fishbone diagram (Figure 2.5).

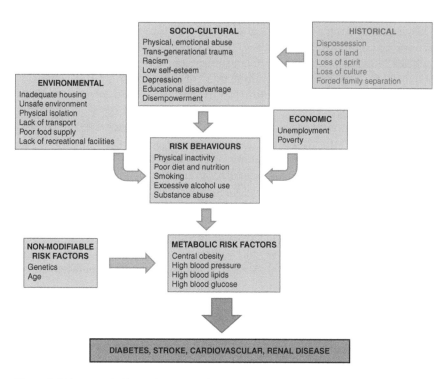

Figure 2.3 Factors influencing vascular health problems among Indigenous Australians.

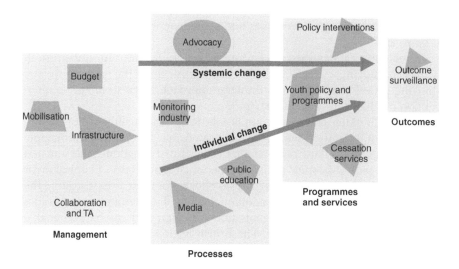

Figure 2.4 Systems thinking approach for addressing tobacco smoking among Indigenous Australian youths.

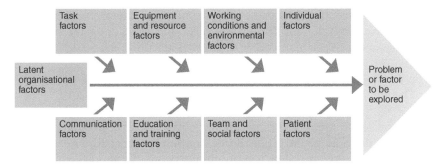

Figure 2.5 'Systems' factors to consider in addressing patient safety issues in hospital settings (adapted from reference 11, p. 158).

Health systems

A Health System may be defined as the structured and interrelated set of all actors and institutions contributing to health improvement. The health system boundaries may then be referred to the concept of health action, which is 'any set of activities whose primary intent is to improve or maintain health'.[12] Health systems expand on the relatively narrow concept of health care systems in the following areas: (1) interrelationships between the components are more useful in gaining understanding and planning interventions than each part examined in isolation; (2) the population is, like the institutional or supply side, an essential part of health systems; (3) ideal health systems value equity, fair financing and responsiveness to legitimate demands of stakeholders; (4) in addition to direct provision of services, health systems function to facilitate stewardship, resource generation and management of health workforce.[13]

The major components of the Australian health system are depicted in Figure 2.6.

Some of the challenges facing Australia's health system were articulated by Professor Jane Hall in a 2010 article:

> the gaps in sub-acute care become evident for the elderly, and those with multiple chronic conditions. This vulnerable group may require more than primary medical care to maintain their health, and once in-hospital may require substantial support for rehabilitation and a return to independent living, or other forms of accommodation. These disjunctions in services are reinforced by funding mechanisms that are service-directed, rather than person-directed; and by poor communication across service streams and across providers. Nonetheless, even in parts of the system that appear to work well, there are problems: problems of unsafe practices and lack of quality; problems of evaluating new technologies before their widespread dissemination; problems of ensuring innovation is

implemented and sustained when warranted; problems in determining and assuring value for the health dollar; and monitoring the performance of the system, particularly in terms of outcomes achieved.[14]

The WHO views health system building blocks as depicted in Figure 2.7. The aims and desirable attributes of the six building blocks are:[15]

1   Good *health services* are those which deliver effective, safe, quality personal and non-personal health interventions to those who need them, when and where needed, with minimum waste of resources.
2   A well-performing *health workforce* is one which works in ways that are responsive, fair and efficient to achieve the best health outcomes possible, given available resources and circumstances. There are sufficient numbers and mix of staff, fairly distributed; they are competent, responsive and productive.

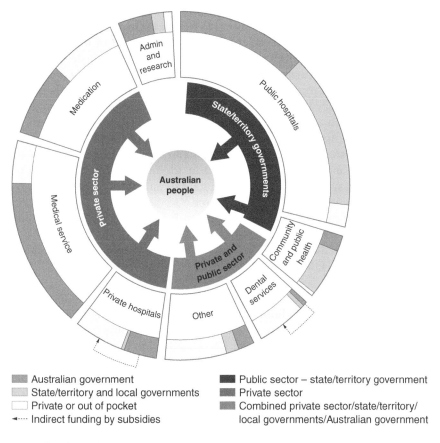

Figure 2.6 Australian health system (adapted from AIHW, Australia Health 2008. Used with permission).

3   A well-functioning *health information* system is one that ensures the production, analysis, dissemination and use of reliable and timely information on health determinants, health systems performance and
health status.
4   A well-functioning health system ensures equitable access to essential
medical products, vaccines and technologies of assured quality, safety, efficacy and cost-effectiveness, and their scientifically sound and cost-
effective use.
5   A good *health financing* system raises adequate funds for health, in ways
that ensure people can use needed services, and are protected from
financial catastrophe or impoverishment associated with having to pay
for them.
6   *Leadership and governance* involves ensuring strategic policy frameworks
exist and are combined with effective oversight, coalition building, the
provision of appropriate regulations and incentives, attention to
system design and accountability.

Health system performance varies widely, even at the same levels of
national income (see Figure 2.8).

The major determinants in variations of health system performance are
leadership, institutions, system design and technologies. Leadership is
perhaps the most critical determinant. It is one of the four main pieces in
the 'New Primary Health Care' jigsaw, as detailed in the 2008 World
Health Report. Katz and Kahn defined leadership as: 'the influential increment over and above mechanical compliance with the routine directives
of the organization'.[16]

Essential leadership activities are summarised in Table 2.1.

The structure and functioning of health-related institutions constitute
a second determinant of health systems. Although public health agencies
are expected to play crucial coordinating and service delivery roles in

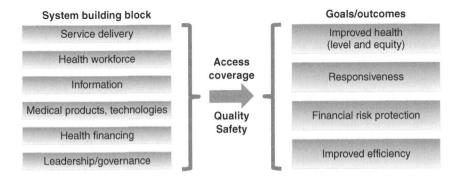

Figure 2.7 World Health Organization's global health system building blocks
(adapted from WHO Health Systems webpage (reference 15)).

Country ratings							
	1.00–2.33						
	2.34–4.66						
	4.67–7.00						
	AUS	CAN	GER	NETH	NZ	UK	USA
OVERALL RANKING (2010)	3	6	4	1	5	2	7
Quality care	4	7	5	2	1	3	6
Effective care	2	7	6	3	5	1	4
Safe care	6	5	3	1	4	2	7
Coordinated care	4	5	7	2	1	3	6
Patient-centred care	2	5	3	6	1	7	4
Access	6.5	5	3	1	4	2	6.5
Cost-related problem	6	3.5	3.5	2	5	1	7
Timeliness of care	6	7	2	1	3	4	5
Efficiency	2	6	5	3	4	1	7
Equity	4	5	3	1	6	2	7
Long, healthy, productive lives	1	2	3	4	5	6	7
Health expenditure/capita 2007	$3,357	$3,895	$3,588	$3,837*	$2,454	$2,992	$7,290

Figure 2.8 Health system performance of selected OECD nations (adapted from the Commonwealth Fund, 2010).

Note
* Estimate. Expenditure shown in $US PPP (purchasing power parity).

health systems, political and socioeconomic factors have weakened public health agencies in many poor countries – e.g. Haiti, Sudan, Afghanistan – to the extent that they are currently marginal contributors to their nations' health systems. The need for long-term investments in the building of health institutions as well as pervasive corruption in the public service of most poor nations have largely discouraged external donors from investing in national health institutions such as Health ministries. Until recently this trend has facilitated the prominence of vertical programmes such as for HIV/AIDS control, with largely negative effects on overall health outcomes not funded under such vertical programmes.[17]

The design of health systems is an important determinant of quality of health care. In Brazil, the implementation (since 1988) of a dynamic, complex, health system design, the Unified Health System – which is based on the principles of health as a citizen's right and the state's duty – has resulted in major gains in health outcomes and efficiency of health care delivery.[18] In contrast, the United States' health system has major inefficiencies due to a poorly designed and over-bureaucratised health system. Major efforts to address design issues through health care reform, such as President Obama's 2010 health care redevelopment initiative, have been stalled on political and ideological grounds. In a March 2001 report, the United States Institute of Medicine (IoM) report, entitled: 'Crossing the quality chasm – a new health system for the

Table 2.1 Major leadership activities

Activity	Definition
Planning and organising	Determine long-term objectives and strategies, allocating resources according to priorities, determining how to use personnel and resources efficiently to accomplish a task or project, and determining how to improve coordination, productivity and effectiveness.
Problem solving	Identifying work-related problems, analysing problems in a systematic but timely manner to determine causes and find solutions, and acting decisively to implement solutions and resolve crises.
Clarifying	Assigning work, providing direction in how to do the work, and communicating a clear understanding of job responsibilities, tasks objectives, priorities, deadlines and performance expectations.
Informing	Disseminating relevant information about decisions, plans and activities to people who need the information to do their work.
Monitoring	Gathering information about work activities and external conditions affecting the work, checking on the progress and quality of the work, and evaluating the performance of individuals and the effectiveness of the organisational unit.
Motivating	Using influence techniques that appeal to logic or emotion to generate enthusiasm for work, commitment to task objectives and compliance with requests for cooperation, resources or assistance; also setting an example of proper behaviour.
Consulting	Checking with people before making changes that affect them, encouraging participation in decision making and allowing others to influence decisions.
Recognising	Providing praise and recognition for effective performance, significant achievements and special contributions.
Supporting	Acting friendly and considerate, being patient and helpful, showing sympathy and support when someone is upset or anxious.
Managing conflict and team building	Facilitating the constructive resolution of conflict and encouraging cooperation, teamwork and identification with the organisational unit.
Networking	Socialising informally, developing contacts with people outside the immediate work unit who are a source of information and support, maintaining contacts through periodic visits, telephone calls, correspondence and attendance at meeting and social events.
Delegating	Allowing subordinates to have substantial responsibility and discretion in carrying out work activities and giving them authority to make important decisions.
Developing and mentoring	Providing coaching and career counselling and doing things to facilitate a subordinate's skill acquisition and career advancement.

21st century'[19] documented health (re)design challenges as shown in Figure 2.9.

The IoM quality in health care report stated in part:

> The fact that more than 40% of people with chronic conditions have more than one such condition argues strongly for more sophisticated mechanisms to coordinate care. Yet health care organizations, hospitals, and physician groups typically operate as separate 'silos,' acting without the benefit of complete information about the patient's condition, medical history, services provided in other settings, or medications provided by other clinicians.[19]

Health care technology is one source of variation in health system performance which is being addressed best so far. There is strong international consensus about effective health technologies, as well as robust global organisations such as GAVI and Global Fund to coordinate equitable delivery of health care technologies. As aptly stated by leading philanthropist Bill Gates in June 2011, during a ceremony in which he and other donors pledged US$4.3 billion to fund vaccine production and delivery to developing nations: 'For the first time in history, children in developing countries will receive the same vaccines against diarrhoea and pneumonia as children in rich countries.[20]

Health systems strengthening is as much about management as it is about resources. As discussed above, despite the United States spending an average of $7,290 per person, its health system performance is

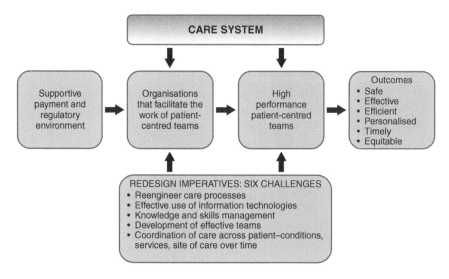

Figure 2.9 Health system redesign challenges in the United States (adapted from IOM Quality Report, 2001).

inferior to the six other Organization for Economic Cooperation and Development (OECD) nations with which it was compared by the Commonwealth Fund in 2007/2008. These nations spent less than half of what the United States spent per person on health care during the review period.[21] In developing nations, money is becoming increasingly less of a constraint for improving the performance of health systems, thanks to the generosity of wealthy nations and private donors. A 2010 report by the Institute of Health Metrics and Evaluation revealed that development assistance for health grew in 2010 to a total of $26.87 billion by year's end, but the rate of growth was cut by more than half from an annual average of 13 per cent between 2004 and 2008 to 6 per cent annually between 2008 and 2010.[22]

Notwithstanding such substantial financial resources, funding for health systems accounts for less than 0.5 per cent of the total annual health expenditure of most developing countries.[23] Efforts to improve the functioning of health systems in developing nations should address the following encumbrances.

Stewardship

Stewardship is an important feature of health governance. It may be described as a political, professional and ethical commitment by health care providers, managers and policy makers to serve the public within its jurisdiction. Accountability for health outcomes is sadly lacking among political and health leaders in developing nations. Also deficient is community/consumer participation in health care. It is important to empower health care consumers such that they have a voice in the management of their local health system.[24]

Regulation

Regulation is best enforced by public health laws/acts. Most developing countries have not adequately revised their public health legislation to address contemporary challenges of health systems. Laws transform the underpinnings of the health system and also act at various points on the complex environments that generate the conditions for health. Those environments include the widely varied policy context of multiple government agencies, such as education, energy and transportation agencies, as well as many statutes, regulations and court cases intended to reshape the factors that improve or impede health. The measures range from national tobacco policy to local smoking bans. Legally enforced public health legislation may be used as interventions in their own right as well as a way to improve health service delivery. Examples include edicts requiring all sex workers in brothels in Thailand to use condoms, and legislation banning the sale of non-iodised salt in China.[25]

Organisational structures and financing

Comparison of organisational structures of health departments in developing and developed nations highlights major deficiencies in the way in which public health agencies are organised (Figures 2.10 and 2.11).

The complexity of health systems in developing nations requires a commensurate organisational structure. For example, there is no formally constituted coordinating body for Non-Governmental Organisations' (NGOs) operations in Uganda's health ministry structure, despite the increasing importance of NGOs in Uganda's contemporary health care system. It may also be appropriate to decentralise some health services management functions, such as giving hospitals and health districts much greater responsibilities for planning and management, and providing hospital and district health system managers with the information, tools and training to enable them to match services and additional resources with the local burden of disease.[26] Financing of health services is compounded by Structural Adjustment Programmes imposed on developing nations as condition for securing loans. For example, until recently, the International Monetary Fund imposed policies that require a public sector 'ceiling' on payroll numbers and salaries thus curtailing the capacity of indebted countries to hire enough health workers or pay them enough to retain them.[27] National health financing systems are equally important, ranging from the percentage of GDP devoted to the health sector, to financing of health insurance and drug revolving funds.

Human resources

In its 2006 World Health report, the WHO estimates that sub-Saharan Africa faces a shortage of more than 800,000 doctors, nurses and midwives and an overall shortage of 1.5 million health care workers, and that a mere 3 per cent of the world's health workers struggle against all odds to combat 24 per cent of the global disease burden.[28] Addressing the shortage requires, among other strategies, encouraging staff retention and motivation through improved remuneration and non-monetary rewards such as opportunities for learning and career progression, subsidised housing and education for dependants, and a culture that values the contribution of health workers.

Ensuring that resource use meets health system objectives

A good starting point for understanding health system objectives is development of consensus on health system functions. The WHO has come up with a list of minimum public health functions that were particularly tailored to the needs of developing nations.[29] Such prioritisation should guide resource allocation. For example, in Papua New Guinea, the top ten diseases that accounted for the most Disability Adjusted Life Years in 2003 are shown in Figure 2.12.

HEALTH AND AGEING ORGANISATIONAL CHART
November 2009

Executive

Secretary — Ms Jane Halton

Deputy Secretary — Ms Mary Murnane

Deputy Secretary — Ms Rosemary Huxtable A/g

Deputy Secretary — Mr Richard Eccles A/g

Deputy Secretary — Mr David Learmouth

Principal Medical Consultant — Prof John Horvath

Chief Medical Officer — Prof Jim Bishop

NHMRC — Prof Warwick Anderson (Independent statutory agency from 1 July 2006)

TGA — Dr Rohan Hammett

NICNAS — Dr Marion Healy

OGTR — Dr Joe Smith

Audit & Fraud Control — Mr Colin Cronin

General Counsel — Mr Chris Reid

Health and Ageing Sector Divisions

Population Health Division — Ms Cath Halbert
- **Office of Health Protection** — Ms Jennifer Bryant
- **Immunisation Procurement Project** — Ms Linda Addison

Primary and Ambulatory Care Division — Ms Jan Bennett

Acute Care Division — Prof Rosemary Calder

Ageing and Aged Care Division — Ms Lesley Podesta
- **Office of Aged Care Quality and Compliance** — Ms Carolyn Smith

Pharmaceutical Benefits Division — Mr Andrew Stuart

Medical Benefits Division — Mr Tony Kingdon

Mental Health and Chronic Disease Division — Ms Georgie Harman
- **Principal Adviser** — Assoc Prof Rosemary Knight

Health Workforce Division — Ms Kerry Flanagan
- **Chief Nurse and Midwifery Officer** — Ms Rosemary Bryant

Cross Portfolio Divisions

Office for Aboriginal and Torres Strait Islander Health — Mr Mark Thomann A/g

Health Reform Taskforce Health — Ms Megan Morris

Portfolio Strategies Division — Ms Linda Powell

Regulatory Policy and Governance Division — Ms Mary McDonald

Business Group — Ms Margaret Lyons; Ms Samantha Palmer; Mr Stephen Sheehan

State/Territory offices

NSW	Ms Gayle Anderson
VIC	Ms Jennifer McDonald
QLD	Ms Elizabeth Cain
ACT	Ms Jackie Stuart-Smith
WA	Ms Nicole O'Keefe
SA	Ms Jan Turbill
TAS	Mr Anthony Speed
NT	Ms Jenny Norris

Figure 2.10 Organisational structure of Australia's Federal Ministry of Health and Ageing (source: CDHA, Canberra 2009).

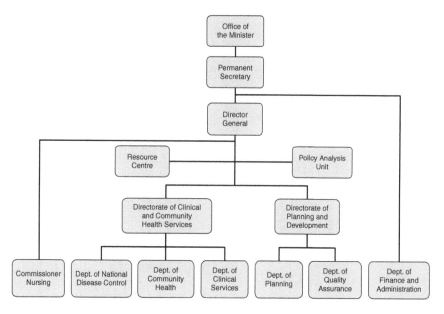

Figure 2.11 Organisational structure of the Ministry of Health, Republic of Uganda (source: Annual Report, MoH, Uganda, 2007).

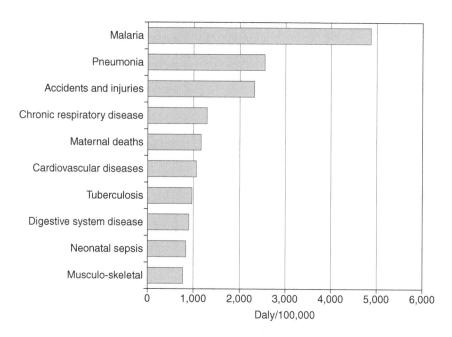

Figure 2.12 Top ten contributors to disease burden in Papua New Guinea, 2003 (adapted from PNG Health Department Report, 2009).

In aggregate, communicable diseases, perinatal, maternal and nutritional causes accounted for 50 per cent of total disease burden and about half of all deaths in Papua New Guinea in 2003. Such data are useful guides in allocation of resources for training, service provision and public education. As organisations and societies become increasingly complex, and as the definition of health is increasingly operationalised by consumers as all-encompassing – with consequent high expectations – the challenges faced by health systems are formidable. Understanding the structure and function of health system is a good starting point for rising to the challenges to be addressed by 'any set of activities whose primary intent is to improve or maintain health'.[12] Another important starting point is a sound theoretical understanding of health organisations, the focus of Chapter 3.

References

1 Mashta, O. New network hopes to define role of health systems in controlling infectious diseases. *British Medical Journal*, 2011; 342: d3156.
2 Preamble to the Constitution of the World Health Organization as adopted by the International Health Conference, New York, 19 June to 22 July 1946; signed on 22 July 1946 by the representatives of 61 states (Official Records of the World Health Organization, no. 2, p. 100).
3 Saracci, R. The World Health Organization needs to reconsider its definition of health. *British Medical Journal*, 1997; 314: 1409.
4 Miles, R.E. The origin and meaning of Miles' Law. *Public Administration Review*, 1978; 38: 399–403.
5 Dolfman, M. The concept of health: an historic and analytic examination. *Journal of School Health*, 1973; 43: 491–497.
6 Becker, M. *The Health Belief Model and Personal Health Behaviour*. Thorofare, NJ: Slack, 1974.
7 Skyttner, L. *General Systems Theory: Problems, Perspectives, Practice*. New York: World Scientific Publishing Company, 2006.
8 Thomson, N., MacRae, A., Burns, J., Catto, M., Debuyst, O., Krom, I., Midford, R., Potter, C., Ride, K., Stumpers, S., Urquhart, B. (2010) *Overview of Australian Indigenous health status, April 2010*. Perth, WA: Australian Indigenous HealthInfoNet.
9 Australian Institute of Health and Welfare. *Substance Use among Aboriginal and Torres Strait Islander People*. Canberra, AIHW, February 2011.
10 Moore, W. *Why Doctors make Mistakes*. London: Channel Four Publications, 2000.
11 National Patient Safety Agency. *Seven Steps to Patient Safety*. London: NPSA, 2003.
12 Murray, C.J.L., Frenk, J. A framework for assessing the performance of health systems. *Bulletin of the World Health Organization*, 2000; 78: 717–731.
13 Frenk, J. The global health system: strengthening national health systems as the next step for global progress. *Plos Medicine*, January 2010; 7(1): 3pp. Available from: www.ncbi.nlm.nih.gov/pmc/articles/PMC2797599/pdf/pmed.1000089.pdf (accessed 20 June 2011).
14 Hall, J. Designing the structure for Australia's health system. Academy of Social Sciences of Australia. Occasional Paper 1/2010.

15 World Health Organization. *Everybody's Business: Strengthening Health Systems to Improve Health Outcomes: WHO's Framework for Action.* Geneva: WHO, 2007.
16 Katz, D., Kahn, R.I. *The Social Psychology of Organisations.* New York: Wiley, 1966.
17 England, R. The dangers of disease specific programmes for developing countries. *British Medical Journal,* 2007; 335: 565.
18 Paim, J., Travassos, C., Almeida, C., Bahia, L., Macinko, J. The Brazilian health system: history, advances, and challenges. *Lancet,* 2011; 377: 1778–1797.
19 Institute of Medicine. *Crossing the Quality Chasm: A New Health System for the 21st Century.* Washington, DC: National Academies Press, 2000.
20 Reuters. Donors pledge $US4.3 billion for vaccines for poor, 13 June 2011. Available from: www.reuters.com/article/2011/06/13/uk-vaccines-donors-idUKTRE75C1FW20110613 (accessed 21 June 2011).
21 The Commonwealth Fund. *National Scorecard on US Health System Performance.* Washington, DC: The Commonwealth Fund, 2006.
22 Institute for Health Metrics and Evaluation. *Financing Global Health 2010: Development Assistance and Country Spending in Economic Uncertainty.* Seattle, WA: IHME, 2010.
23 Mills, A., Rasheed, F., Tollman, S. Strengthening Health Systems. In *Disease Control Priorities in Developing Countries,* 2nd edn, eds Jamison, D.T., Breman, J.G., Measham, A.R., Alleyne, G., Claeson, M., Evans, D.B., Jha, P., Mills, A., Musgrove, P., 87–102. New York: Oxford University Press, 2006.
24 Berlan, D., Shiffman, J. Holding health providers in developing countries accountable to consumers: a synthesis of relevant scholarship. *Health Policy and Planning,* 2011; 1–10: b doi:10.1093/heapol/czr036.
25 Institute of Medicine. *For the Public's Health: Revitalizing Law and Policy to meet New Challenges.* Washington, DC: National Academy of Sciences, 2011.
26 Nyonato, F.K., Awoonor-Williams, K., Phillip, J.F., Jones, T.C., Miller, R.A. The Ghana community-based health planning and services initiative for scaling up service delivery innovation. *Health Policy and Planning,* 2005; 20: 25–34.
27 Buckley, R.P., Jonathon, B. IMF policies and health in Sub-Saharan Africa. In *Global Health Governance: Crisis, Institutions and Political Economy,* eds Kay, A., Williams, O., London: Palgrave Macmillan, 2008. Available from: http://law.bepress.com/unswwps/flrps08/art14/ (accessed 30 March 2012).
28 World Health Organization. *World Health Report 2006: Working Together for Health.* Geneva: WHO, 2006, pp. 8, 12–13.
29 Bettcher, D.W., Sapirie, S., Goon, E.H. Essential public health functions: results of the international Delphi study. *World Health Statistical Quarterly,* 1998; 51: 44–54.

3   Theories of health organisations

Health systems-related theories

The word theory is derived from the Greek word *Theoria*, and it was originally defined as beholding or contemplation, as opposed to practice. It has over time become increasingly obvious that the distinction between theory and practice is not as extreme. A more appropriate contemporary definition of theory was provided by van Ryn and Heany: 'systematically organized knowledge applicable in a relatively wide variety of circumstances devised to analyse, predict or otherwise explain the nature or behaviour of a specified set of phenomena that could be used as the basis for action'.[1] Theories are structured logical explanations with the following characteristics:

- an integrated set of propositions that serves as an explanation for a phenomenon;
- introduced after a phenomenon has already revealed a systematic set of uniformities;
- a systematic arrangement of fundamental principles that provide a basis for explaining certain happenings of life.

Theories have enabled humans to develop an understanding of their environment since the ascendancy of community life. The earliest theories about creation and our place as humans in the universe facilitated the evolution of organised religion. Theories of creation ranged from the biblical account in Genesis, through sacred anthills in Hinduism to the Rainbow Serpent in Indigenous Australian spirituality.[2] Philosophical reasoning challenged creationist paradigms by questioning the evidence for its assumptions. For example, Spinoza's ethical injunction for the intellectual states: 'Do not deplore, do not laugh, do not hate, but understand.'[3] Models explaining creation from non-spiritual perspectives were provided by Hans Sloane, who focussed on environmental factors,[4] and Robert Chambers, who proposed the transmutation model of species diversity.[5] Charles Darwin was able, through painstaking observations during his

extensive voyage around South America and Australia, as well as application of evolution models based on the ideas of Sloane, Chambers and
comparative anatomy to propound his theory of evolution through natural
selection in 1859.[6] This theory was built upon to formulate evolution
frameworks based, among others, on theories of continental drift, asteroid
blast, and climate change.[7] Thus, theories serve as important links between
models and frameworks (Figure 3.1).

Theories play important roles in facilitating the objectives of health
organisations. In the health promotion sector, for example, Hochbaum *et
al.* describe theories as statements and relationships identifying factors
that are likely to produce particular results under specified conditions[8]
Good health promotion theories, skilfully adapted, can help predict what
consequences interventions are likely to have, even in novel situations.
Examples of health promotion theories, and their appropriate contexts,
are shown in Table 3.1.

As shown in Table 3.1, there are several broad categories of health promotion theories: theories explaining health behaviour change in individuals, theories explaining change in communities, theories explaining
change in organisations and theories explaining the development of
healthy public policy.

Concept of organisations

The word 'organisation' is derived from the Greek word *Organon* – a com-
partment for a particular job. Organisations are social and legal arrangements within which individuals structurally interact to pursue collective
goals. Organisations strive to adapt, control their performance and have

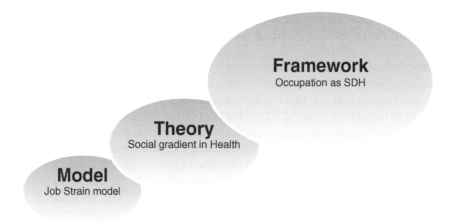

Figure 3.1 Relationship between models, theories and frameworks – author's
perspective.

Table 3.1 Using context-specific theories to predict health behaviour

	Theory	Focus	Key concepts
Individual level	Stages of Change Model	Individual's readiness to change or attempt to change towards healthy behaviours	Pre-contemplation Contemplation Decision/determination Action Maintenance
Interpersonal level	Social Learning Theory	Behaviour is explained via a 3-way, dynamic reciprocal theory in which personal factors, environmental influences and behaviour continually interact	Behaviour capability Reciprocal determinism Expectations Self-efficacy Observational learning Reinforcement
Community level	Community Organisation Theories	Emphasises active participation and development of communities that can better evaluate and solve health and social problems	Empowerment Community competence Participation and relevance Issue selection Critical consciousness

physical or imaginary boundaries separating them from their environments. Modern organisations are characterised by: planned relational and
behavioural patterns – standardisation and formalisation; a structure of
roles – organogram, job descriptions; planned procedures, policies and
strategic objectives, understood as specific structures; everyday interactions
(social actions) of organisational members – i.e. the informal
organisation.

Organisations are the building blocks of systems or institutions. Institutions may be defined as 'a social collectivity distinguished by primacy of
orientation to the attainment of a specific goal or goals'.[9] Differences (and
relationships) between organisations and institutions are summed up
thus:

> Institutions are patterned ways of dealing with recurrent social issues
> and establish an environment within which organisations operate.…
> Organisations, by contrast, are structures of social relationship, social
> actors arranged in positions and roles; usually, but not always, deliber-
> ately arranged and designed to achieve some end or ends. Organisa-
> tions are distinct from institutions by being arrangements of roles and
> positions. Such organisational relationships are regulated by norms
> which are deliberately constructed to achieve a specified goal.… Insti-
> tutions shape organisations by providing a normative context within
> which organisations seek their ends. Organisations reproduce institu-
> tions by conforming to their norms and from time to time seek to
> change institutions. Institutions provide a normative context both lim-
> iting and facilitating social change.[10]

In the capacity building context, systems and institutions are coterminous.
Health organisations derive from two main institutions. The mental health
organisations evolved from the punishment institution, and until the past
two centuries in most of Europe, mental asylums and prisons were
managed using similar organisational structures.[11] Most other health
organisations evolved from the social institutions of religion and charity.[12]
The tension between health organisations and the social institutions is
inherent in current efforts to reformulate basic health care provision as a
human right rather than a charity.[13]

Most organisations are characterised by value patterns or structures.
Ideally, values held by individuals are expected to be congruent with those
of organisations with which they are affiliated, but this is not always the
case. Values that organisations espouse, or more accurately are espoused
on their behalf by senior managers can, in some cases at least, reflect
organisational practices, and in most or all cases, they reflect what senior
managers actually believe their organisations to be like, what they would
like or prefer their organisations to be like, or what they would like significant stakeholders to believe the organisation is like.[14]

Organisational values define the acceptable standards which govern the behaviour of individuals within the organisation. Without such values, individuals will pursue behaviours that are in line with their own individual value systems, which may lead to behaviours that the organisation doesn't wish to encourage. In New South Wales, Australia, 'Public Health Organisation' is defined by the Health Services Act 1997 as an Area Health Service, statutory health corporation and an affiliated health organisation in respect of its recognised establishments and recognised services. The Vision of New South Wales Justice Health organisation is: 'International best practice health care for those in contact with the criminal justice system.' The values of Justice Health are equitable access, client centred services, professionalism, accountability and transparency, evidence-based practice, collaboration, forward thinking.[15]

Health organisations may be distinguished by many criteria, including spatial scope (e.g. international, national or local), size (e.g. small, medium or large), ownership (e.g. public, private or not for profit) and function (e.g. clinical, public health or research). These categorisations enable comparative studies of function and structure of health organisation.[16] Health organisations are complex, adaptive systems. Improvement of health care organisations individually and collectively, and research on those organisations, will be best facilitated by comprehensive application of the metaphor of the system as a living organism, rather than the system as a machine. This perspective has implications for the choice of theories for use in health organisations, given the business/industrial origins of most commonly used theories of health organisations, at least until recent decades.[17,18]

Health organisations are so diverse structurally and functionally that it is usually difficult to study them in a coherent way, or to apply findings from one organisation to another. However, shared learning is precisely what is required if modern health organisations are to function efficiently.[19] As stated by Val Moore, Implementation Programme Director of the UK's National Institute for Clinical Excellence (NICE) in January 2011 while publicising the 2011 Shared Learning awards:

> The aim of the Shared Learning Awards is to recognise and reward organisations who have actively tried to find new ways of working to implement NICE guidance and ultimately improve health and wellbeing for patients and their families or the broader public ... some examples may not have worked brilliantly at every stage or produced large scale results, but that doesn't matter. The awards are a platform for organisations to share their stories so that others can learn from them.[20]

Organisational theories help to highlight common features of organisations which may be studied to guide interventions such as capacity building. The commonly used organisational theories in health are the focus of the next chapter.

Theories of health organisations

'Whenever a theory appears to you as the only possible one, take this as a sign that you have neither fully understood the theory, nor the problem which it was intended to solve.'[21] A well-developed theory of organisations may be described as a systematically (logically)-related set of propositions expressing relationships between the 'elements' of organisations – properties or characteristics such as their size, efficiency, degree of centralisation and complexity. Organisational theory may be defined as the study of organisations for the benefit of identifying common themes for the purpose of solving problems, maximising efficiency and productivity, and meeting the needs of stakeholders. Broadly, organisational theory can be conceptualised as studying three major subtopics: individual processes, group processes and organisational processes.[22]

Health organisations are characterised by a wide diversity of forms and structures, but are characterised by the overarching vision of creating the conditions in which people may be healthy. They are also characterised by the shared adaptation of organisational theories, which fall under three broad groups: classical theories, human relations theories and systems theories. This section discusses several theories in each of these groups, and their implications for the management of health organisations.

Classical theories. Max Weber (1864–1920) is generally regarded as the 'Father of Organisational Theory'. His most enduring contribution to organisational management is his theory of bureaucracy. He framed the overriding task of bureaucracy as determining how it can achieve the purpose and mission of organisations with the greatest possible efficiency and at the least cost of any resources. Bureaucratisation was, for Weber, the key part of the rational-legal authority and a key process in the ongoing rationalisation of the Western society. He characterised effective bureaucracies as having: (a) fixed division of labour; (b) hierarchy of offices; (c) rational-legal authority; (d) specified performance measures; (e) selection based on qualifications; (f) clear career paths.[23]

Weber's vision of an 'ideal types' bureaucracy is characterised by formal training for the performance and coordination of specific organisational tasks. It takes time and experience to learn the job, not so much because it is difficult to perform the particular task, but because it all has to be coordinated. Modern bureaucracies typically seek educated recruits. Their education will be attested by some certificate, since bureaucracies prefer operating with impersonal criteria and 'objective' evidence. Weber speaks of 'credentialism', the preoccupation evident in modern societies with formal educational qualifications. While credentialism has been effective to a large extent in influencing the quality of staff employed in health organisations, it has also created complexity and reduced flexibility in task shifting for frontline workers in health care organisations.[24] Given the global health care worker shortage, bureaucratic bottlenecks need to be addressed if task shifting and other health workforce innovations are to be effectively deployed to address health workforce shortage in developing nations (Figure 3.2).[25]

Mintzberg[26] described health care organisations as professional bureaucracies, as opposed to 'machine' or classical bureaucracies found in most business sectors and the majority of government departments. Professional bureaucracies are characterised by specialist departmental line staff having a large measure of control over the content of work by virtue of their professional knowledge and skills. Hierarchical directives issued by those nominally in control of health care organisations (e.g. non-clinical directors of public health units) often have limited impact in influencing organisational culture and practices. This may result in organised anarchy, with too many leaders and too few followers and consequent dispersion of organisational vision. Professional bureaucracies in less developed countries thus typically suffer from a lack of horizontal integration, with overlaps and functional deficiencies in health coverage, leading to poor financial accessibility to care, marked heterogeneity in the quality of care and an absence of quality assurance mechanisms. Mintzberg

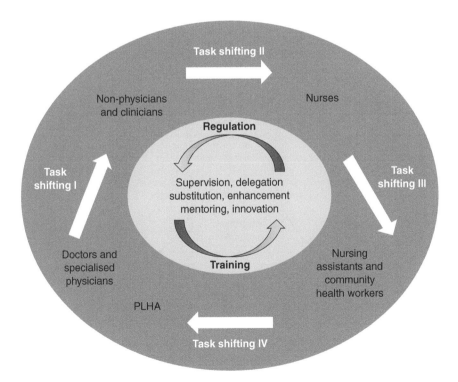

Figure 3.2 Task shifting in health organisations addressing HIV/AIDS (adapted from WHO Health Systems Task Shifting Booklet, 2007).

distinguished five components of an organisation: the strategic apex, the techno-structure, an operational core, the supporting staff and the middle line. This schema may be adapted to National Health Service organisations,[27] although it is noteworthy that Mintzberg paid inadequate attention to community participation, an important process in the efficient functioning of modern health organisations (Figure 3.3).

Another classical theorist whose influence in health care organisations remains remarkable is Frederick Taylor, who proposed a theory of 'scientific management' of organisational tasks, which he claimed to improve employee efficiency and organisational performance. His theory's principles are:[28] (i) develop a science of work by measuring optimal output, skills, workforce and machine requirements; (ii) scientific selection of workers with the right aptitude for specific jobs and their adequate training, educating workers and management about the benefits of scientific management, and specialisation and collaboration between workers and management (Figure 3.4).

Taylor's theory of scientific management derives from Positivist models. His work was strongly influenced by the social and historical period in which he lived. His lifetime (1856–1915) was during the Industrial

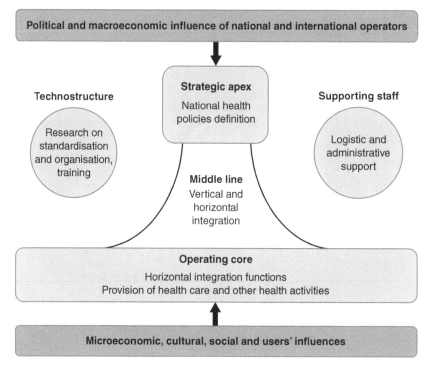

Figure 3.3 Mintzberg's adaptation of five components of organisational to health ministries (adapted from reference 27).

Revolution. The overall industrial environment of this period is well documented by Dickens' classic novel, *Hard Times*. Autocratic/mechanistic management was the norm. However, health organisations are complex adaptive systems which are not nearly as influenced by the predictability of industrial processes.[29] Positivist models view organisations as machines and people as appendages to such machines. Although still a feature of 'sweatshop' units within health organisations (e.g. some patient care assistants and laboratory workers), Taylor's theory of 'production first, people second' is generally unsuitable for complex modern health organisations.

Human relations theories. Human relations theories are normally thought of as having their roots in the Hawthorne Studies conducted in the 1920s and 1930s at the Hawthorne works of the Western Electric Company, near Chicago in the United States. Elton Mayo and his team demonstrated, to some extent, the importance of 'the human factor' in organisations. He advocated for workers to be recognised as having social needs and interests such that they could no longer be regarded as the economically motivated automatons envisaged by Taylorism. Interestingly, the 'lightning studies', which involved varying light intensity in workstations, were associated with productivity increases in both study and control groups. This finding suggested that what the researchers were doing was of interest and importance to the workers. It was this which caused the increase in productivity and which demonstrated that the workers could not be regarded as mere parts in the organisational machine – the 'Hawthorne Effect'. This principle has been applied in health care settings, where doctors, under observation by researchers, deliver patient care services at a higher quality compared with when unobserved.[30]

Abraham Maslow (1908–1970) theorised that:[31] (1) people have different needs and therefore need to be motivated by different incentives to achieve organisational objectives; (2) people's needs change over time, meaning that as the needs of people lower in the hierarchy are met, new needs arise. Maslow suggests that if organisational leaders want to motivate

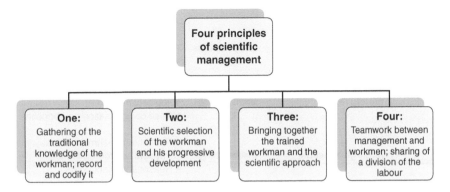

Figure 3.4 Taylor's principles of scientific management.

participants, they need to know where within the hierarchy such participants are placed. He suggested that competitive salary will address physiological needs, and safe work conditions will address safety needs. His
hierarchy of needs, and organisational management implications, are rep-
resented in Figure 3.5.

Maslow's theory has received little empirical support especially in relation to the hierarchical structure of needs. It was also difficult to prove a
causal relationship or consistent correlation between need and behaviour.
For example, former BP Chief Executive Tony Hayward stated several
times in reports in May 2010; 'I want my life back', during clean-up efforts
of the oil spill in the Gulf of Mexico. Such statements imply 'lower-order
needs', and directly contradict Maslow's hierarchy approach. This theory
is particularly unsuitable for professional bureaucracies such as health
organisations where the majority of frontline participants are educated to
tertiary level and are keen to succeed, but are also keen to have internationally competitive salaries.

Another management theorist whose contributions to health organisations have been remarkable is Renesis Likert. He posited that the more
the job is supervised, the less productive the workers. He outlined four
systems of management to describe the relationship, involvement and
roles of managers and subordinates in organisational settings. He urged
organisations to work towards 'integrative unity' – extensive interaction,
friendly work environment and high levels of trust (Table 3.2).

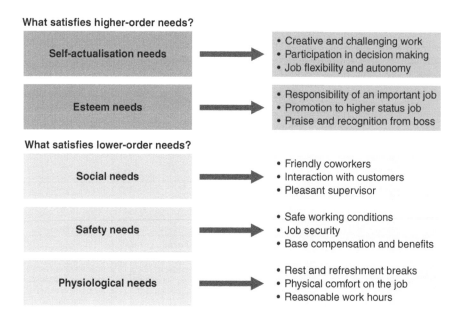

Figure 3.5 Maslow's hierarchy of needs – organisational management implications.

Table 3.2 Likert's Trust–Motivation–Interaction grid

	Trust	Motivation	Interaction
System 1	No trust	Fear, threats and punishment	Little interaction, always distrust
System 2	Master/servant	Rewards and punishment	Little interaction, always caution
System 3	Substantial but incomplete trust	Rewards, punishment, some involvement	Moderate interaction, some trust
System 4	Complete trust	Goals based on participation and improvements	Extensive interaction, friendly, high trust

Likert contrasted exploitative management system (I) with participative group systems (IV), and endorsed the latter as the most productive. However, a deficiency of Likert's HR management theory is that over-identification with (or over-reliance on) groups may conflict with organisational objectives, and encourage 'Groupthink'. 'Professional' health bureaucracies are particularly susceptible to devolving into disconnected hierarchies and Groupthink. Also many important causes of job satisfaction and organisational cohesiveness in health organisations (e.g. organisational commitment)[32] lie outside Likert's organisational management grid. He appeared to be focussed on positive management outcomes, but provided little guidance on how such outcomes may be achieved in complex organisations.

Systems theories. In this context the word *systems* is used to refer specifically to entities that are self-correcting through feedback. Self-regulating systems are found in nature, including the physiological systems of our body, as well as in organisations. Health organisations exemplify complex adaptive systems, defined as: 'a collection of individual agents who have the freedom to act in ways that are not always totally predictable, and whose actions are interconnected such that one agent's actions change the context for other agents'.[33] New structures and forms of behaviour emerge that cannot be obtained by summing the behaviours of the constituent parts, because new system properties emerge from the nonlinear interactions between agents. The diversity, extent, intricacy and strength of the relationships influence the system's ability to adapt. There may be too much connectivity in some parts of the system, as well as too little interaction relative to need in others.[34]

Eric Trist pioneered studies on the role of professional cultures, ergonomics and social attitudes in organisational dynamics. In 1949, he found that technological developments had enabled Yorkshire coal miners to work in small autonomous groups, with each person responsible for a range of tasks, rather than the highly specialised and routinised production-line approach then common in industry. He showed that improved worker autonomy, participatory decision making processes and harmonisation of organisational cultures with technology optimise organisational cohesion and productivity. This research has become known as the sociotechnical systems approach, and it had considerable impact on the way work is organised (Figure 3.6).[35]

Trist's theory of organisation asserts that organisational change efforts that combine coordinated social and technical interventions stand a greater chance of success than either might result in if initiated separately. Strongly linked with this goal has been the development of a theory of work design that is based on the study of the whole work system, organised in terms of self-regulating groups and multi-skilled individuals. Important features of sociotechnical systems include variety, learning opportunity, own decision power, organisational support and social recognition. His findings remain relevant in many fields of modern health organisations, such as ergonomics.[36]

Activity Theory, as developed by Finnish educationist Yrjo Engestrom (1987), is a means of analysing organisational processes. In a 1987 study, he found organisational pressure on GPs from four sides: (1) bureaucracies: rule adherence vs patient satisfaction; (2) patients: more time per patient vs shorter waiting periods; (3) nurses: teamwork vs independence from physicians; (4) specialists: early screening vs restricted GP referrals.[37] Engestrom argued that contradictions in organisational structures and objectives give rise to 'need states', hence a need for organisational change in order to satisfy emerging needs. For example, new policies were required in Finland to choose one element of the contradiction over the other: 'patients as life systems' must take precedence over 'patients as quantity' (object contradiction); 'rules of cost-effectiveness' must yield to 'rules of prevention' (rules contradiction) – Figure 3.7.[37] He determined that new forms of work organisation result from resolving contradictions, and increasingly require negotiated 'knotworking' across boundaries.

A basic area of convergence of organisational theories is role specificity. All theorists ascribe to role specificity, but to varying degrees. Weber posits

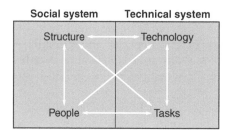

Figure 3.6 Eric Trist's sociotechnical systems approach.

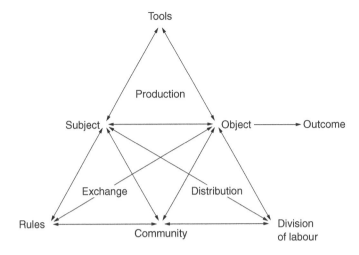

Figure 3.7 Engestrom's activity sub-systems of a Finnish primary care centre (adapted from reference 37).

that high role specificity, as in rational-legal bureaucracies, lead to higher performance. Likert suggests that low role specificity is more ideal for modern organisations, as this stimulates innovation. However, lower role specificity may cause anxiety when staff are not able to rely on detailed guidance from management. Activity Theory may be utilised to address such contradictions.

Choice of theory for health organisations should reflect compatibility between a theory's assumptions and the values of the group where the theory will be used to inform an intervention. Managers of modern health organisations require theories that may facilitate interventions that are patient centred, as well as politically, fiscally, socioculturally and administratively feasible. In health organisations, a need exists for 'home-grown' health organisation theories, which are custom designed for the realities of health care delivery settings. Sir Michael Marmot's Theory of Social Gradient of Disease[38] is exemplary. Finally, health organisations need to invest in organisational development, not just leadership development. This will entail strengthening the role of all staff as followers. The above theories provide guideposts for effective organisational development.

References

1 Van Ryn, M., Heaney, C.A. What's the use of theory? *Health Education Quarterly,* 1992; 19: 315–330.
2 Irwin, J.C. The sacred anthill and the cult of the primordial mound. *History of Religions,* 1982; 21: 339–360.

3 Spinoza, B. *Ethics* (1677). New York: Everyman Classics, translation by G.H.R. Parkinson, 1989.
4 Morrison, E. The collection of natural history specimens in Jamaica 17th–19th century. Jamaica Clearing House Mechanism, March 2007.
5 Chamber, R. *Vestiges of the Natural History of Creation*. London: John Churchill, 1844.
6 Darwin, C. *On the Origin of Species by Means of Natural Selection, or the Preservation of Favoured Races in the Struggle for Life*. London: John Murray, 1859.
7 Parmesan, C. Ecological and evolutionary responses to recent climate change. *Annual Review of Ecology and Evolutionary Systems*, 2006; 37: 637–669.
8 Hochbaum, G.M., Sorenson, J.R., Lorig, K. Theory in health education practice. *Health Education and Behaviour*, 1992; 19: 295–313.
9 Parsons, T. *Structure and Process in Modern Societies*, New York, Free Press, 1960, p. 17.
10 Bouma, G. Distinguishing institutions and organisations in social change. *Journal of Sociology*, 1998; 34: 232–245.
11 Goffman, E. *Asylums: Essays on the Social Institution of Mental Patients and other Inmates*. New York: Doubleday, 1961.
12 Quandagno, J. Institutions, Interest Groups, and Ideology: an agenda for the sociology of health care reform. *Journal of Health and Social Behavior*, 2010; 51: 125–136.
13 Kickbusch, I. From charity to rights: proposal for five action areas for public health. *Journal of Epidemiology and Community Health*, 2004; 58: 630–631.
14 Kabanoff, B, Daly, J. Espoused values of organisations. *Australian Journal of Management*, 2002; 27: 89–105.
15 Justice Health. *Annual Report 2007/2008*. Sydney: NSWHEALTH, 2008.
16 Ramanujam, P.G. Service quality in health care organisations: a study of corporate hospitals in Hyderabad. *Journal of Health Management*, 2011; 13: 177–202.
17 Alderson, P. The importance of theories in health care. *British Medical Journal*, 1998; 317: 1007–1010.
18 Borowski, N. *Organizational Behaviour, Theory, and Design in Health Care*. Sandbury: John & Bartlett Publishers, 2009, pp. 428–432.
19 Atkins, J.M, Walsh, R.S. Developing shared learning in multi-professional health care education: for whose benefit? *Nursing Education Today*, 1997; 17: 319–324.
20 National Institute for Health and Clinical Excellence. Final call for entries for NICE's Shared Learning Awards. London: NHS 13 January 2011. Available from: www.nice.org.uk/newsroom/news/FinalCallForEntriesForNICEsSharedLearning Awards.jsp (accessed 24 June 2011).
21 Popper, K. *Conjectures and Refutations: The Growth of Scientific Knowledge*. London: Routledge & Kegan Paul, 1963.
22 Crombie, A. The case study method and the theory of organisations. *Journal of Sociology*, 1969; 5: 111–120.
23 Weber, M. *The Theory of Social and Economic Organization*. London: Collier Macmillan Publishers, translation by A.M. Henderson and T. Parsons, 1947.
24 Tyler, W. Complexity and control: the organisational background of credentialism. *British Journal of Sociology of Education*, 1982; 3: 161–172.
25 World Health Organization. Task shifting to tackle health worker shortages. Geneva: WHO, WHO/HSS/2007.03, 2007.
26 Mintzberg, H. *The Structuring of Organisations*. Englewood Cliffs, Prentice-Hall, 1979.
27 Unger, J., Macq, J., Bredo, F., Boelaert, M. Through Mintzberg's glasses: a fresh look at the organization of ministries of health. *Bulletin of the World Health Organization*, 2000; 78(8): 1005–1014.

28 Taylor, F.W. *The Principles of Scientific Management.* New York: Harper & Brothers, 1919.

29 Plsek, P., Wilson, T. Complexity, leadership, and management in healthcare organisations. *British Medical Journal,* 2001; 323: 746–749.

30 Leonard, K.L. Is patient satisfaction sensitive to changes in the quality of care? An exploitation of the Hawthorne effect. *Journal of Health Economics,* 2008; 27(2): 444–459.

31 Schwartz, H. Maslow and the hierarchical enactment of organisational reality. *Human Relations,* 1993; 36: 933–956.

32 Al-Hussami, M. A study of nurses' job satisfaction: the relationship to organizational commitment, perceived organizational support, transactional leadership, transformational leadership, and level of education. *European Journal of Scientific Research,* 2008; 22: 286–295.

33 Plsek, P., Greenhalgh, T. Complexity science: the challenge of complexity in health care. *British Medical Journal,* 2001; 323: 625–628.

34 Sibthorp, B., Glasgow, N., Longstaff, D. *Complex adaptive systems.* Australian National University: Australian Primary Health care Research Institute, 2004.

35 Ramage, M., Shipp, K., Trist, E. *Systems Thinkers.* London: Open University Press, 2009, Ch. 29).

36 Carayon, P., Smith, M.J. Work organization and ergonomics. *Applied Ergonomics,* 2000; 31: 649–662.

37 Engestrom, Y. *Learning by Expanding: An Activity-Theoretical Approach to Developmental Research.* Helsinki: Orienta-Konsultit, 1987.

38 Marmot, M. Historical perspective: the social determinants of disease – some blossoms. *Epidemiological Perspectives and Innovations,* 2005; 2: 4.

4 Structures and functions of health organisations

Structural evolution of health organisations

Health organisations evolved as separate units from society's social structure from about the late seventeenth century. Prior to this period, the health provider, or shaman, was invariably a leading political and religious figure. Hence, health care provision religion and political leadership were intricately linked. The organisations that provided health services prior to the seventeenth century were thus structured along religious lines, but with strong political support. For example, in medieval Europe, religious organisations operated as health organisations in establishing leper colonies throughout Europe. Segregation of leprosy was justified on religious grounds, and missionaries provided charity to 'sinful' residents of leprosaria.

In societies in which monotheistic religion has not developed, shamans or medicine men were also religious leaders and health care providers. In shamanistic religions, a medicine is some magical object or ceremony, such as a medicine bag, that is used to control and direct supernatural forces. Among the North American Indians, a medicine man or medicine woman is someone who professes to have skills at manipulating supernatural forces and uses these skills to cure sickness, drive away evil spirits and regulate the weather. Medicine items attributed with various supernatural abilities for the bag would often be procured in a tribal custom known as a vision quest. This ceremony includes personal sacrifice: fasting and prayer over several days in a location isolated from the rest of the community, often involving hallucinogens. The purpose was to make contact with natural spiritual forces that help or guide people to reach their potential. The spirits or totems would aid the individual to gather magical items, increase knowledge and aid personal growth.[1]

The next phase in the evolution of health organisation was the ascendancy of medicine. In 1896, Edward Jenner was able to demonstrate that vaccination, albeit a crude version, protected against smallpox, a major public health problem at the time. Although Edward Jenner is credited with the development of vaccination, it was first introduced into England by Lady Mary Wortley Montague in 1721. She tried a method that was used in Turkey where people deliberately infected themselves with a mild form of smallpox. Nevertheless, the widely publicised findings of Edward Jenner created a medical renaissance, and facilitated the transfer of authority from religious leaders and shamans to doctors in relation to the development of health organisations.[2] There was also a significant correlation between poverty reduction and evolution of hospitals. In 1929, the British Local Government Act was promulgated. This Act abolished the boards of guardians who administered the Poor Laws and gave local authorities the prerogative to convert Poor Law workhouses into municipal hospitals, thereby making indoor as well as outdoor medical relief more readily available.[3]

It is noteworthy that the prominence of medicine in the development of health organisations did not include the mental health sector, which evolved as part of the punishment institution, a process detailed by Foucault in *Madness and Civilisation*.[4] The non-mental health sector developed by physicians evolved along the lines of Christian care centres. Hospices (originally called xenodochia), initially built to shelter pilgrims and messengers between various bishops, developed into hospitals in the modern sense of the word. As scientific origins of diseases were discovered, the evolving medical profession developed sub-specialities such as apocathery, whose practitioners prepared therapeutic medications, a role reserved for the pharmacist today. In its investigation of herbal and chemical ingredients, the work of the apothecary may be regarded as a precursor of the modern sciences of chemistry and pharmacology, prior to the formulation of the scientific method.

The hospital as the centrepice of health organisations created significant problems for patients and caregivers. Limited knowledge of the pathogenesis of disease led to high rates of nosocomial infections. During the Crimean war (1853–1856), Florence Nightingale worked in a military hospital, and showed that 80 per cent of soldiers died from infections they caught in the hospital rather than their original wounds. Florence Nightingale improved standards of hygiene and sanitation which dramatically reduced the infections in her hospital. When she returned from the war, Florence Nightingale embarked on a campaign to modernise and improve hospitals. She set the foundations of hospital organisation and establishment of nursing as a formal health profession.[5] Efforts to improve and modernise hospital management as the centrepiece of modern health organisations were largely unsuccessful, due in part to the medical hegemony, limited utilisation of reflective practice and resistance to ideas for reform. For example Ignaz Semmelweis' study of the relationship between doctors' hand washing practices and puerperal mortality in the 1840s (Figure 4.1) was ignored or rejected by the medical establishment for decades for ideological rather than scientific reasons.[6]

The next phase in the evolution of health organisations was commenced with the passage of the 1948 Public Health Act in England and Wales, which set up General Boards of Health to provide mainly sanitation and infection control services.[7] Local Boards of Health were authorised to appoint employees such as surveyor, inspector of nuisances, clerk, treasurer and an officer of health (who had to be a qualified doctor). The main focus of the health boards was environmental sanitation, with particular reference to sewers, street cleansing, public toilets, slaughter houses, street paving, recreation parks, water supply and burials. The headship of public health boards by medically qualified staff strengthened all public health's links to health organisations, thus broadening its scope.

By 1948, another milestone in the evolution of health organisations was initiated in the United Kingdom with the establishment the British National Health Service (NHS). The doctors were determined to maintain their lucrative private practice and keep their distance from medical officers of health and post-war discussions on what they perceived as a 'socialist' health service being foisted on the nation by then Labour Party health minister Aneurin Bevan. Following substantial concessions, doctors provided conditional cooperation for the NHS on 28 May 1948, and the NHS became a reality on 5 July 1948.[8]

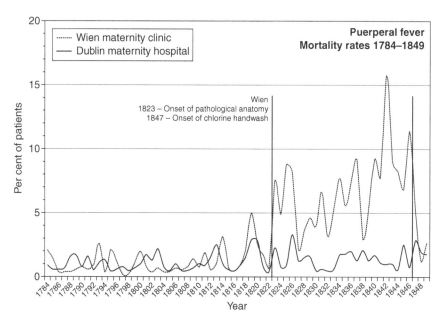

Figure 4.1 Semmelweis' 1881 book which compared rates of puerperal fever in Wien Hospital (Vienna) and Dublin Hospital (Ireland) prior to onset of pathological anatomy and chlorine hand wash (source: Wikipedia (public domain). Available from: http://en.wikipedia.org/wiki/File:Yearly_mortality_rates_1784–1849.png (accessed 29 March 2012)).

The NHS provided a template for the organisation of health services in the Western world. Also, colonised nations in Africa, Asia and Latin America adopted the NHS model of centralised, hospital-centred, doctor-led national health services. However, a different model of health care organisation was evolving in China and, to a lesser extent, the former Soviet Union. This model focused on utilising community health workers to provide low cost primary health services as close as possible to where people lived. In China, a 'barefoot doctors' programme was commenced in 1968 as a national policy focused on quickly training community health workers to meet basic rural health needs. Most 'barefoot doctors', who graduated from secondary school education, practised after training at the county or community hospital for three to six months. Hence, medical coverage in the countryside rapidly expanded. This programme served as a catalyst for similar training programmes in many developing nations. In addition, the British organisational concept of building general and tertiary hospitals was challenged by oriental organisational structures based on comprehensive health centres which provided day-care and outreach services, and which complemented relatively few general and tertiary hospitals. The Chinese and Soviet 'low cost' initiatives were adopted as global framework for health care organisations with the Alma Ata declaration of 1978. Unfortunately, while the Alma Ata declaration conceptualised primary health care as an approach to health care development, powerful critics framed it as merely the first level of care.[9] This controversy limited the Primary Health Care model's global impact on health care organisation.

Health care reform also facilitated important changes in health care organisations. In the United Kingdom, the first major reorganisation of the NHS since its inception in 1948 took place on 1 April 1974, the aim of which was to 'provide a fully integrated service in which every aspect of health care could be provided by the health professions'. This reform of the NHS was formulated in line with the politicians' and policy makers' perspective at that time that a bio-psychosocial model of health care organisation is a better organisational framework compared with the bio-medical approach. A series of organisational changes followed in the areas of clinical accountability and responsible autonomy, to redress a situation described by former chief medical officer of the Scottish Department of Health, Sir John Brotherston, as 'syndicalistic anarchy' – excessive freedom by the medical profession at the expense of organisational cohesion. These changes exerted major influence in the NHS such that by 2005, its organisational structure was significantly less dominated by physicians (Figure 4.2).[10,11]

Other important influences on health organisation globally include the health promotion movement, which facilitated the positioning of non-medically qualified public health workers as equal partners with medical practitioners, economic restructuring programmes with health impacts

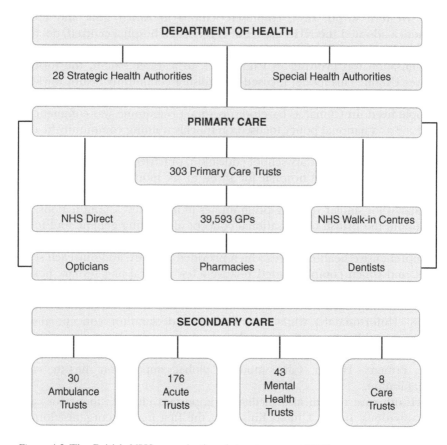

Figure 4.2 The British NHS organisational structure as at 2005.

such as the privatisation drive for health services as part of structural adjustment programmes and the revitalisation of primary health care with its strong social justice and human rights values. Currently, mergers, integration, decentralisation, private–public partnership and downsizing, all of which may include changes in work assignments, modifications to clinical staffing and skill mix, and reductions in management positions, are increasingly common in modern organisations. These changes have important implications for the structure of modern organisations.

Structures of modern health organisations

There are many ways of describing organisational structures. For example, the structures may vary in relation to government funding, as public, private and not for profit organisations. Organisational structure may also vary in size, resulting in classifications such as small, medium and large health organisations. In this section, the author describes health organisation structure in relation to scope, as international, national and local health organisations. One example is utilised for health organisations at each level.

International health organisations

The World Health Organization (WHO) is perhaps the best known international health organisation. WHO can be considered the primary agency of the United Nations that promotes global public health. It was founded on 7 April 1948. Its responsibilities include: providing leadership on matters critical to health and engaging in partnerships where joint action is needed; shaping the research agenda and stimulating the generation, translation and dissemination of valuable knowledge; setting norms and standards and promoting and monitoring their implementation; articulating ethical and evidence-based policy options; providing technical support, catalysing change and building sustainable institutional capacity; and monitoring the health situation and assessing health trends.[12]

WHO, like many other international organisations, has a complex, albeit decentralised organisational structure. The headquarters is based in Geneva, Switzerland, and there are about 8,100 staff in six regional offices located in 147 individual country offices. The importance of this structure lies in the fact that the regional offices can focus on health matters that are of concern in their particular region and can act as a liaison with their local country offices to further develop and implement policies. In contrast, the headquarters is concerned with more general matters that are likely to affect all parts of the world (4.3).

The organisational human resources framework operates on a cluster approach, with teams of five to 25 staff working on projects. For example, the Health Systems and Services Cluster programmes focus on essential medicines, ethics, equity, trade and human rights, health financing and social protection, health policy and service delivery, human resources for health, blood safety, laboratories and health technology.[13] Project teams working on different clusters report to departmental directors, while groups of departmental directors report to the Assistant Director General. Assistant Directors General report to the Director General, currently Dr Margaret Chan. Clusters are usually moved across departments when organisational changes occur. For example, on 21 November 2007, Dr Chan announced that the Health Technology and Pharmaceuticals cluster, which includes the departments of Essential Health Technologies, Medicines Policy and Standards and the department of Technical Cooperation for Essential Drugs and Traditional Medicine, will be restructured and merged into the Health Systems and Services cluster in recognition of the fact that 'access to safe, effective, affordable medicines and other technologies is a fundamental component of an effective health system'.[14]

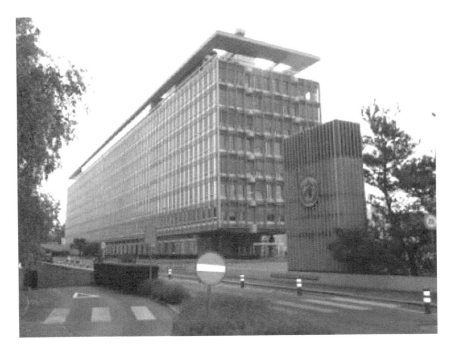

Figure 4.3 Office of the World Health Organization, Geneva.

At the regional level of WHO, organisational structures vary depending on health priorities. The WHO Regional Office for Africa is located in Brazzaville, Republic of Congo. The Regional Office is headed by the WHO Regional Director for Africa, who is elected for a period of five years. The operations of the Regional Office are decentralised through three Inter-country Support Teams (ISTs) based in Harare, Libreville and Ouagadougou. The 46 WHO Country Offices and WHO Liaison Offices support countries in reaching their national health goals and in contributing to global and regional public health action.

The '70–30 per cent' principle continues to guide the overall distribution of resources between front-line WHO workers in countries (70 per cent of total budget), regional offices and WHO headquarters, as directed by the strategy of strengthening first-line support to countries while ensuring adequate back-up from headquarters and the regional offices (30 per cent of total budget). The total 2010–2011 operating budget of WHO is US$3.368 billion, a reduction of 10 per cent relative to 2008–2009, but comparable to the 3.3 billion expended during the 2006–2007 financial year. On average, member states provide 28 per cent of the funding, with the remaining 72 per cent coming from a diverse range of voluntary contributors such as other UN organisations, foundations and the private sector.[15]

National health organisations

The National Aboriginal Community Controlled Health Organisation (NACCHO) is the national peak Aboriginal health body representing Aboriginal Community Controlled Health Services (ACCHSs) throughout Australia. An ACCHS or an Aboriginal Medical Service (AMS) is a primary health care service initiated and operated by the local Aboriginal community to deliver holistic, comprehensive and culturally appropriate health care to the community which controls it (through a locally elected board of management). There are currently 141 ACCHSs in Australia. Formed in 1976, NACCHO remains an important organisation for community health capacity building in Indigenous settings. The organisational structure is shown in Figure 4.4.

Membership of NACCHO is open to Aboriginal community controlled health services that have met the NACCHO criteria for membership. The membership criteria into NACCHO are determined by state or territory peak Aboriginal community controlled health bodies affiliated with NACCHO. They include:

i   Local Aboriginal Community controlled as defined by the Organisation's Rules;
ii commitment and adherence to the NACCHO definition of Aboriginal Health as defined by the Organisation's Rules;
iii culturally appropriate;

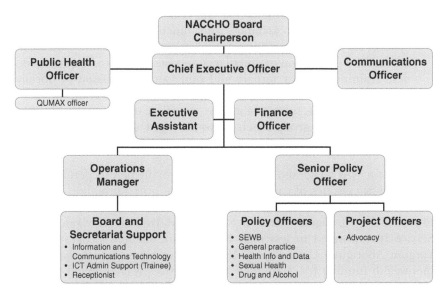

Figure 4.4 Organisational structure of NACCHO.

iv   an incorporated local Aboriginal Community controlled organisation
     operating an Aboriginal Health Service; and
v   providing primary health care.

NACCHO's main roles include formulating memoranda of understanding
and partnership agreements with stakeholders, political advocacy, workforce development, support for development of ACCHSs, management of
Aboriginal health data, drafting discussion and position papers, and
health governance. NACCHO advocates that all ACCHSs should be
funded and supported to provide integrated comprehensive primary
health care and that the services listed below should constitute integrated
comprehensive primary health care:

> Primary clinical care such as: treatment of illness using standard treat-
> ment protocols; 24 hour emergency care; provision of essential drugs;
> management of chronic illness; Population health/preventive care
> such as: immunisation; antenatal care; appropriate screening and
> early intervention (including adult and child health checks and sec-
> ondary prevention of complications of chronic disease); communica-
> ble disease control; Clinical support systems such as: pharmaceutical
> supply system; a comprehensive health information system (popula-
> tion registers, patient information recall systems, and systems for
> quality assurance); Staff training and support such as Aboriginal
> health worker training, cross cultural orientation, continuing educa-
> tion; Management systems that are adequately resourced, financially
> accountable and include effective recruitment and termination prac-
> tices; Adequate infrastructure at the community level such as staff
> housing and clinical facilities, and functional transport facilities;
> Systems for supporting visiting specialists and allied health profession-
> als, medical evacuation or ambulance services; access to hospital facili-
> ties; Training role for tertiary and other students; Based on locally
> relevant priorities and the availability of funds for programs directed
> at rheumatic fever, substance misuse, nutrition, environmental health,
> particular target groups such as youth, aged and disabled people;
> Support for the community on local, state and federal issues.[16]

Funding for NACCHO and its agencies is generally tied to performance,
measured as episodes of care. ACCHSs provide over 1.6 million episodes
of care yearly. Annual funding varies from about $8 million for big centres
like Redfern Aboriginal Medical Service and Derbarl Yerrigan Health
Service Incorporated to less than $750,000 for smaller services such as
Yorgum Aboriginal Corporation. About 75 per cent of Australian Commonwealth funding for Aboriginal health services is channelled through
NACCHO/ACCHSs. The government's 2007–2008 budget of $526.2
million is primarily allocated to funding health service providers for the

delivery of primary health care services to their local communities (~$374 million) and funding new programmes and services through new budget measures (some of which are directed at facilitating access to primary health care services and increasing the uptake of the Medicare Benefits Schedule/Pharmaceutical Benefits Scheme (~$150 million).[17] NACCHO was largely successful in its 2008 advocacy for increased funding of Indigenous health programmes to the tune of $1.84 billion over four years[18] – the Australian government announced new funding of $1.6 billion for NACCHO over four years in 2009.

Local health organisations

The first successful local government in Australia was established in Melbourne in 1842. Currently, considerable variations exist in local government size and structure. For example, in the state of New South Wales (NSW), there are currently 176 local government councils. The largest council is Blacktown City Council with a population of over 244,000 people and an area of 241 km². The smallest NSW council is Hunters Hill Municipal Council with a population of just over 13,000 people and a land area of just 6 km². Local governments in Australia do not have a constitutional responsibility for health. However, they perform essential sanitation and other health functions as delegated by the state health departments, in accordance with state public health acts. In Tasmania, for example, the state's Public Health Act 1997 requires councils to: (a) develop and implement strategies to promote and improve public health; (b) ensure that the provisions of this Act are complied with; and (c) carry out any other function for the purpose of this Act that the Minister or Director determines. In relation to water supplies, the Act specifies that each council must monitor the quality of water within its municipal area in accordance with any relevant guidelines (s. 130). The Director may require a council to carry out a health evaluation of water under its management or control (s. 132).[19]

In Western Australia, Armadale City Council health unit exemplifies a local health organisation. The City of Armadale is the suburban local government representing the communities of Armadale, Bedfordale, Brookdale, Camillo, Champion Lakes, Forrestdale, Haynes, Hilbert, Kelmscott, Karragullen, Mt Nasura, Mt Richon, Roleystone, Seville Grove and Wungong. The municipality spans 545 km² and has an estimated population of 55,000. Armadale City Council is made up of 14 Councillors, including the Mayor. Elections are held every two years, with seven of the 14 Councillors participating at any one time. Council meets regularly to make decisions on behalf of local residents. All local issues are divided into one of four distinct areas. They are City Strategy, Development Services, Technical Services and Community Services. Health issues generally fall under the Development Services portfolio (Figure 4.5).

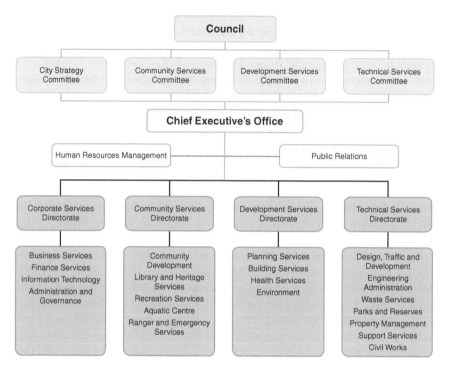

Figure 4.5 Organisational structure of Armadale City Council (adapted from Armadale Council Corporate Structure Website).

The Armadale Council's Development Services Directorate is responsible for the following health-related areas: planning and development; town planning schemes; land use; environment; building and health control; noise control; immunisation; signage. In addition, the Western Australia health department has delegated the management of the following child health centres to Armadale Council: Armadale Child Health Centre, Challis Child Health Centre, Kelmscott Child Health Centre, Roleystone Child Health Centre, Westfield Child Health Centre, Wungong Child Health Centre.

The human resources infrastructure of most local government public health units appear inadequate to address the considerable functions delegated to it. Indeed, it is possible to link most local government activities with public health activities such as in Table 4.1.

Vaccination is one area where most Australian local governments fall short. A majority of local governments lack adequate immunisation nurses, hence their contributions to state-wide children vaccination programmes remain sub-optimal. For example, records obtained from selected local governments councils in Queensland on their contributions to children's immunisation in 2004 are shown in Table 4.2. Thus, there appears to be a

Table 4.1 Public health-related functions of local governments in Australia

- Provision of a safe potable water supply
- Removal, treatment and management of solid and liquid waste
- Ensuring healthy housing and accommodation
- Mosquito control
- Control of vermin
- Control of nuisances including animals, dust, noise, overgrown lots, smoke and fumes
- Safety of noxious and hazardous goods
- Prevention of infectious disease
- Ensuring food safety
- Regulation of personal appearance services (hair dressing, skin penetration)
- Management of sharps
- Management of recreational waters including public pools/spa
- Street cleaning
- Immunisation
- Control of mass events
- Public health planning and promotion
- Environmental pollution response and cleanup
- Protecting health in disasters and emergencies

mismatch between organisational structure and organisational functions in relation to public health at most Australian local government councils.

Functions of health organisations

Civil society organisations

While, structurally, health organisation functions may be conveniently divided into local, national and international organisations, from a functional perspective, health organisation functions may be viewed from the perspectives of civil society organisations (CSO), public health organisations and public–private health partnerships. The WHO Director General emphasised the need to consider the three organisational sectors in health improvement in her 2007 World Health Day message:

> Given the growing complexity of these health and security challenges and the response required, these issues concern not only governments, but also international organizations, civil society and the business community. Recognizing this, the World Health Organization is making the world more secure by working in close collaboration with all concerned.

The World Bank defines CSOs as:

> The wide array of non-governmental and not-for-profit organizations that have a presence in public life, expressing the interests and values

of their members or others, based on ethical, cultural, political, scientific, religious or philanthropic considerations. Civil Society Organizations (CSOs) therefore refer to a wide array of organizations: community groups, non-governmental organizations (NGOs), labor unions, indigenous groups, charitable organizations, faith-based organizations, professional associations, and foundations.[20]

The number of internationally operating CSOs is estimated at 40,000. National numbers are even higher: Russia has 277,000 CSOs; India was estimated to have around 3.3 million NGOs.[21] At a global level, CSOs such as the International Baby Food Action Network (IBFAN) have been

Table 4.2 Vaccination profiles of the 30 (out of a total of 120) Queensland councils that provide vaccination services

Council	Not immunised 2003/2004 aged <8	Population 2002	% population immunised 2003/2004
Barcaldine Shire Council	230	1,732	13.3
Beaudesert Shire Council	29	55,612	0.1
Brisbane City Council	9,967	917,216	1.1
Bundaberg City Council	194	45,043	0.4
Caboolture Shire Council	388	116,992	0.3
Esk Shire Council	75	14,869	0.5
Fitzroy Shire Council	127	10,010	1.3
Gladstone City Council	157	27,099	0.6
Gold Coast City Council	1,233	438,473	0.3
Hervey Bay City Council	1,199	44,402	2.7
Ipswich City Council	1,823	128,986	1.4
Jondaryan Shire Council	14	13,229	0.1
Kilkivan Shire Council	10	3,227	0.3
Kingaroy Shire Council	100	11,990	0.8
Kolan Shire Council	14	4,672	0.3
Logan City Council	200	169,433	0.1
Longreach Shire Council	279	4,033	6.9
Mackay City Council	305	77,157	0.4
Maryborough City Council	865	25,260	3.4
Miriam Vale Shire Council	8	4,620	0.2
Mount Isa City Council	2,507	20,785	12.1
Murweh Shire Council	280	5,030	5.6
Nanango Shire Council	40	8,540	0.5
Pine Rivers Shire Council	1,657	127,439	1.3
Redland Shire Council	475	120,371	0.4
Rockhampton City Council	1,076	59,410	1.8
Sarina Shire Council	55	9,862	0.6
Toowoomba City Council	1,157	91,187	1.3
Warwick City Council	136	21,387	0.6
Winton Shire Council	257	1,611	16.0
	24,857	2,579,677	1.0

Source: Queensland immunisation records, 2003/2004.

instrumental in developing an international code for the marketing of breast milk substitutes which was adopted by the WHO member states in May 1981.[22] The campaign by IBFAN and other CSOs in mounting a boycott of the leading food manufacturer Nestlé, in protest against its marketing practices promoting formula milk as healthier than breast milk, was highly successful at drawing worldwide public attention to the health consequences arising from such practices, and for creating a code of practice against which the actions of food manufacturers could be assessed. Civil society groups are also active in AIDS and breast cancer activism locally, nationally and internationally.[23,24]

The health-related functions of CSOs include issues linkage, agenda setting, advocacy, translational research, monitoring and evaluation, standardisations of norms and procedures, policy analysis and implementation, capacity building and financing. CSOs are also becoming increasingly political, as evidenced by their involvement in recent uprisings in North Africa, which led to changes in leadership in Egypt and Tunisia in the first half of 2011. In Australia, CSOs were instrumental in getting Indigenous health disadvantage to national consciousness. CSOs such as Save the Children, Australian Council of Social Services and Oxfam established a national Close the Gap Day, lobbied governments, developed a National Close the Gap Equality targets document as an advocacy tool, and provided key policy input into the governments' strategies for addressing Indigenous disadvantage.[25] At an international level, CSOs have remained actively involved in global health governance and global health issues including poverty alleviation and debt relief for impoverished nations. The Global Call to Action Against Poverty is an umbrella organisation of scores of CSOs who advocate for poverty alleviation policies globally, especially during their annual White Band Day marches. The world Hepatitis Alliance, an NGO focused on raising public awareness and funding for people afflicted with viral hepatitis, recently secured WHO endorsement of the first annual World Hepatitis Day on 28 July 2011. The theme for the 2011 Day was 'Hepatitis affects everyone, everywhere. Know it. Confront it.' Viral hepatitis constitutes a significant public health problem in most nations and, in some, such as Egypt, which has 10 per cent of its population living with hepatitis C, and Vietnam, where adult prevalence of hepatitis B is about 15 per cent, such functions of CSO enable stakeholders to use information about viral hepatitis and stimulate effective and sustainable interventions.

Public health organisations

Public health organisations exist primarily to discharge public health functions. Public health functions continue to evolve with the expanding scope of public health. By 1852 when the first international sanitary conference was held in Paris, public health functions were essentially sanitary functions. The modern public health movement has a set of minimum functions, defined as; 'indispensable set of actions, under the primary responsibility of the state, that are fundamental for achieving the goal of public health which is to improve, promote, protect, and restore the health of the population through collective action'.[26] Pan American Region WHO's 11 essential public health functions (EPHF) are:

EPHF 1 – Monitoring, evaluation, and analysis of health status

EPHF 2 – Surveillance, research, and control of the risks and threats to public health

EPHF 3 – Health promotion

EPHF 4 – Social participation in health

EPHF 5 – Development of policies and institutional capacity for public health planning and management

EPHF 6 – Strengthening of public health regulation and enforcement capacity

EPHF 7 – Evaluation and promotion of equitable access to necessary health services

EPHF 8 – Human resources development and training in public health

EPHF 9 – Quality assurance in personal and population-based health services

EPHF 10 – Research in public health

EPHF 11 – Reduction of the impact of emergencies and disasters on health

These functions have been incorporated into the national public health development strategy and public health training programmes of most developing countries. For example, in Costa Rica, efforts have been made to strengthen EPHF 8 (human resources development) through the characterisation of the public health workforce at the national and regional levels as well as in urban and rural areas. In Mexico, a major effort to improve EPHF 8 has been made by the Veracruzana University through the implementation of a new curriculum for its Master of Public Health Programme, entirely based on the EPHF. The goal of the programme is to form graduates that will become professionals committed to the development of the EPHF.

Wealthy nations have worked to develop their country-specific public health functions. In the United States, three core public health functions are assessment, policy development, and assurance. These core functions are linked to ten essential services. *Assessment:* (1) monitor health status to identify community health problems; (2) diagnose and investigate health problems and health hazards in the community; (3) evaluate effectiveness, accessibility and quality of personal and population-based health services. *Policy development* (4) develop policies and plans that support individual and community health efforts; (5) enforce laws and regulations that protect health and ensure safety; (6) research for new insights and innovative solutions to health problems. *Assurance* (7) link people to needed personal health services and assure the provision of health care when otherwise unavailable; (8) assure a competent public health and personal health care workforce; (9) inform, educate and empower people about health issues; (10) mobilise community partnerships to identify and solve health problems.[27] In Australia, the public health functions were agreed upon in 1999 following a national survey. The functions were broadly similar to those of the WHO and the United States. Importantly, the study also determined functions which were not generally regarded as public health functions in Australia (Table 4.3).[28]

A list of essential public health is useful in streamlining definitions and prioritisation of public health activities, such as capacity building, expenditure mapping and development of performance standards. Other potential uses of determining a list of public health functions for specific settings include defining public health functions more clearly, determining the capacity required to deliver public health functions, assessing whether this capacity currently exists and building public health capacity where required.

The evaluation utility of public health functions is well exemplified by their use to evaluate the Indian public health system. The research utilised the WHO EPHFs to evaluate public health practices in India. The evaluation report stated:

> India has relatively poor health outcomes, despite having a well-developed administrative system, good technical skills in many fields, and an extensive network of public health institutions for research, training, and diagnostics. This suggests that the health system may be misdirecting its efforts, or be poorly designed ... The data indicate that the reported strengths of the system lie in having the capacity to carry out most of the public health functions. Its reported weaknesses lie in three broad areas. First, it has overlooked some fundamental public health functions such as public health regulations and their enforcement. Second, deep management flaws hinder effective use of resources, including inadequate focus on evaluation; on assessing quality of services; on dissemination and use of information; and on openness to learning and innovation. Resources could also be much better utilized with small changes, such as the use of incentives and challenge funds, and greater flexibility to reassign resources as priorities and needs change. Third, the central government functions too much in isolation and needs to work much more closely with other key actors, especially with sub-national governments, as well as with

Table 4.3 Items attracting the least support as public health functions in Australia

	Always a public health function (core)	Often a public health function	Sometimes a public health function	Not a public health function
8 Prevention, surveillance and control of non-communicable disease				
8.5 Provision of anti-depressant drugs	2.8	12.5	40.3	44.4
8.4 Provision of cholesterol lowering and anti-hypertensive drugs	8.3	9.7	51.4	30.6
8.6 Drug treatment and rehabilitation services (e.g. methadone)	12.5	26.4	45.8	15.3
8.3 Chronic disease self-management	16.7	22.2	48.6	12.5
10 Health growth and development programmes and services				
10.7 Prevention-based care from alternative or complementary therapists	2.7	12.3	49.3	35.6
10.6 Individual medical check ups	4.1	15.1	45.2	35.6
10.5 Individual dental check ups	6.8	15.1	46.6	31.5
10.2 Prenatal and neonatal screening	26.1	27.5	34.8	11.6
2 Ensuring healthy and safe environments				
2.5 Controlling land degradation and soil loss (e.g. by erosion)	15.1	23.3	46.6	15.1
2.8 Ensuring access to facilities for social interaction	20.8	25.0	40.3	13.9
2.6 Ensuring access to public transport and educational opportunities	19.4	29.2	40.3	11.1

Source: adapted from Australia Public Health Functions (Delphi) survey, 1999.

the private sector and with communities. We conclude that with some re-assessment of priorities and better management practices, health outcomes could be substantially improved.[29]

Hospitals and 'clinical' organisations

Hospitals and organisations involved with direct provision of patient care comprise a variety of workers, ranging from volunteers to highly skilled health professionals. Core functions of modern hospitals include: diagnosing and treating diseases, surgery for patients requiring an operation; medicines from government dispensaries; training of interns and other students in medicine, nursing and allied health; immunisation for children against many preventable diseases; family planning and maternity care; and emergency care to victims of accidents and disasters. These functions have evolved over time. Hospital's historical meaning was 'a place for hospitality', particularly for strangers, and they were established around the eighth century by nuns to care for the poor, serve as accommodation for travellers and as schools for training staff in care and hospitality. Until the second half of the twentieth century, mental hospitals were the most prominent source of patient care. Mental hospitals met multiple needs of patients – treatment, care, shelter and asylum.[30] Hospitals represent the main concentration of resources and health professional skills in health systems. They are often viewed as rivals to public health or community health services. This antithesis is false, but widely believed, in part due to the erroneous perception that primary health care is a level of health care, when in fact it is an orientation to health care that includes a well-functioning hospital system (Figure 4.6).

Hospitals also sub-serve non-core but important functions, such as providing status for communities in which they are situated, reinforcing the pre-eminence of curative/clinical medicine in health care services and serving as a focus point for volunteers who help to provide services and raise funds. Hospitals are increasingly being run as business organisations. The commodification of health care has important implications for the cost of health care services to patients and government, as well as in the development of public–private partnerships. Narrowly focussed hospital expansion, especially following the end of the Second World War, resulted in physicians developing a disease model of health care, and in the setting up of vertical disease control programmes which functioned not only for service provision, but also for prestige and profit.

Internationally, the coordination of hospital functions is primarily through the International Hospital Federation (IHF). IHF is the global association of health care organisations, which includes in particular, but not exclusively, hospital associations and representative bodies as well as their members and other health care related organizations. The role of the IHF is to help international hospitals work towards improving the level

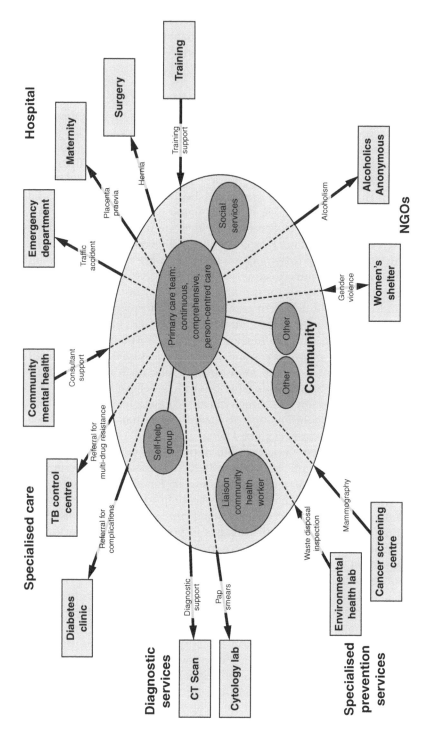

Figure 4.6 Primary health care as an orientation to health care, with hospitals playing a pivotal role.

of the services they deliver to the population regardless of that population's ability to pay. The IHF recognises the essential role of hospitals and health care organisations in providing health care, supporting health services and offering education. The IHF is a unique arena for all major hospital and health care associations to cooperate to act upon their critical concerns. Current IHF projects include Fighting Multidrug Resistant Tuberculosis, Infant and Child Food Safety Program, Mobility of Health Professionals Project and the Corporate Leadership Council.[31]

References

1 Important.ca. Shamanism and medicine. Available from: www.important.ca/index.html (cited 13 July 2010).

2 Riedel, S. Edward Jenner and the history of smallpox and vaccination. *Baylor University Medical Center Proceedings*, 2005; 18: 21–25.

3 Wilson, N. *Municipal Health Services*. London: Allen and Unwin, 1946.

4 Foucault, M. *Madness and Civilization: A History of Insanity in the Age of Reason*. New York: Vintage-Random House, translated by R. Howard, 1988.

5 Arstein, M.G. Florence Nightingale's influence on nursing. *Bulletin of the New York Academy of Medicine*, 1956; 32: 540–546.

6 Nuland, S.B. The enigma of Semmelweis: an interpretation. *History of Medicine and Allied Sciences*, 1979; 34: 255–272.

7 Krieger, N., Birn, A. A vision of social justice as the foundation of public health: commemorating 150 years of the spirit of 1848. *American Journal of Public Health*, 1998; 88: 1603–1606.

8 Honigsbaum, F. The evolution of the NHS. *British Medical Journal*, 1990; 301: 694–699.

9 Bryar, R. Primary health care: does it defy definition? *Primary Health Care Research and Development*, 2000; 1: 1–2.

10 DHSS. *Management Arrangements for the Re-organised Health Service: The Grey Book*. London: HMSO, 1972.

11 Department of Health. *A Patient-led NHS*. London: HMSO, 2005.

12 World Health Organization. *Working for Health: An Introduction to the World Health Organization*. Geneva, Switzerland: WHO, 2007.

13 WHO. *Health Systems & Services Cluster: Programmes and Organizational Structure*. Geneva: WHO, 2011.

14 WHO media centre. More changes in WHO structure announced. Media Centre, 21 November 2007.

15 WHO. *Proposed programme budget 2011–2012*. Geneva: WHO Director-General, 2009.

16 National Community Controlled Aboriginal Health Services. Official website. Available from: www.naccho.org.au/definitions/acchs.html (accessed 20 July 2011).

17 Australian Government Office of Evaluation and audit (Indigenous programs). *Evaluation of Primary Health Care Funding to Aboriginal and Torres Strait Islander Health Services*. Canberra: Australian Government, 2009.

18 National Aboriginal Community Controlled Health Organisation. *Budget Submission 2008/09*. Canberra: NACCHO, 2008.

19 Government of Tasmania. Public Health Act 1997: an Act to protect and promote the health of communities in the State and reduce the incidence of preventable illness. Hobart, Tasmania, 1998.

20 World Bank. *Defining Civil Society*. Washington, DC: World Bank, 2010. Available from: http://web.worldbank.org/WBSITE/EXTERNAL/TOPICS/CSO/0,,con tentMDK:20101499~menuPK:244752~pagePK:220503~piPK:220476~theSiteP K:228717,00.html (accessed 25 July 2011).

21 World Bank. *Civil Society Organizations*. Washington, DC: World Bank Group. Available from: http://web.worldbank.org/WBSITE/EXTERNAL/TOPICS/CS O/0,,contentMDK:20127718~menuPK:288622~pagePK:220503~piPK:220476~t heSitePK:228717,00.html (accessed 29 March 2012).

22 World Health Assembly. International Code on Marketing of Breastmilk Substitutes, WHA Resolution 34.22. Geneva, WHA, 1981.

23 Goldstein, S., Usdin, S., Scheepers, E., Japhet, G. Communicating HIV and AIDS, what works? A report on the impact evaluation of Soul City's fourth series. *Journal of Health Communication*, 2005; 10: 465–483.

24 Alan, R.A., Bell, S.E. Artworks, collective experience and claims for social justice: the case of women living with breast cancer. *Sociology of Health and Illness*, 2007; 29: 366–390.

25 Awofeso, N. The 2008–2030 National Indigenous Health Equality Targets: suggestions for transforming potential into sustainable health improvements for Indigenous Australians. *Australian Indigenous Health Bulletin*, 2010; 10 (2). Available from: http://healthbulletin.org.au/wp-content/uploads/2010/04/bulle-tin_original_articles_awofeso.pd (accessed 29 March 2012).

26 World Health Organization. *Essential Public Health Functions as a Strategy for Improving Overall Health Systems Performance*. Geneva, WHO, 1997.

27 Centers for Disease Control and Prevention. *National Public Health Performance Standards Program*. Atlanta: CDC, 2006.

28 National Public Health Partnership. *National Delphi Study on Public Health Functions in Australia*. Melbourne: NPHP, 2000.

29 Das Gupta, M., Rani, M. India's public health system: how well does it function at the national level? World Bank Policy Research Working Paper 3347, November 2004.

30 Parsons, T. The mental hospital as a type of organization. In *The Patient and the Mental Hospital*, eds Greenblatt, M., Levinson, D.J., Williams, R., 108–129. Glencoe, IL: Free Press, 1957.

31 International Hospital Federation. Official website. Available from: www.ihf-fih.org/ (accessed 17 August 2011).

Part II

Management of health organisations

5 Management prescribed, observed and interpreted

If you ask managers what they do, they will most likely tell you that they plan, organise, co-ordinate and control. Then watch what they do. Don't be surprised if you can't relate what you see to those four words.

Henry Mintzberg

Management is tasks. Management is discipline. But management is also people. Every achievement of management is the achievement of the manager. Every failure is the failure of the manager. People manage, rather than forces or facts. The vision, dedication and integrity of managers determine whether there is management or mismanagement.

Peter Drucker

Management prescribed, managers observed

As with the literature on organisations, much of the literature on management is prescriptive, being more concerned with telling us what managers should do rather than describing and explaining what managers actually do. Prescriptive approaches are characteristic of the instrumental accounts of management. In these accounts, managerial work was depicted as being rational and goal-directed and composed of neutral, technique-based processes whose use, it was claimed, would enhance managers' capacity to direct organisations as instruments for goal attainment. As discussed in Chapter 2, management is variously presented as comprising a series of technical tasks informed by objective science in the case of Scientific Management, or as a socially ameliorative process informed by applied social science in human relations theory. In systems theory, management is seen as being composed of systems maintenance functions.

For scientific management writers, management encompassed the following depersonalised, technical tasks: planning, organising, directing, staffing, coordinating, reporting, budgeting ('PODSCORB'), scheduling, designing and dividing work. Writers such as Henri Fayol and Frederick Taylor argued that there were efficient and inefficient ways of going about these tasks. The efficiency with which each of the tasks was performed depended on the task centredness and objectivity of the manager concerned and the degree to which, in doing his/her work, she/he made use of what were claimed to be scientifically based techniques whose effectiveness had been proven. Human relations writers emphasised the social dimensions and responsibilities of management and in so doing, extended discussion beyond the technical tasks and routines of 'PODSCORB'. Management was presented in terms of its leadership functions with respect to building the social climate of the organisation, ensuring the affiliation of organisational participants, providing not only work but social support to workers and engendering conditions of work, both physical and social, in which workers can develop to their full potential. Systems theorists emphasised the systems maintenance functions of management arising from the open systems characteristics of organisations which made these prone to a wide range of internal and external forces. Thus management was presented as a neutral, technical and socially enabling process which centred on maintaining a balance amongst environmental, technical and human factors and hence on maintaining the organisation as a functioning system. Contingency theorists rejected the notion that it was possible to identify a series of universal principles for management. Rather, they saw the effectiveness of individual managerial strategies as being situation-bound; some strategies being more appropriate in some situations than others.[1]

The question; 'what do managers actually do?' has an air of naivety, even redundancy to it, given that it is a common consensus that the quality of management is critical to the achievement of organisational outcomes. Such notions presuppose that managerial contributions to organisational outcomes are identifiable, measurable and tangible. Studies of managerial work by Mintzberg[2] and studies of managerial behaviour by Stewart,[2] have helped to illuminate managerial activities. Apart from survey approaches, case study approaches have also been useful in learning more about day-to-day activities of managers. When viewed from a political perspective, it is readily apparent that 'management' is not a single entity and certainly not a single-minded one. Managers have been shown to be participants in continuing contests characterised by contingent power and shifting coalitions.[3] The pervasiveness and centrality of managerial politics in organisations has been aptly summarised by Palumbo:[4]

> When organizations are viewed as political systems, budgets become annual treaties; reorganizations are indicators of ruling coalition changes, and decision rules reflect existing internal alliances. There is even an analogy to international relations in that much inter-organizational contact is direct toward the 'forging of alliances', which not only furthers the interests of the participants but also creates a powerful 'network of influence'. Such alliances may be open; they may also be secret. The key to organizational (managerial) behaviour,

then, lies in a description of the processes which attend the distribution of power and the actors involved. Within a medical school, contests frequently occur between physicians and researchers; in a corporation, between production and sales; in a health agency, between health officers, nurses and sanitarians.

Recognition of the full scope of politics in organisational life (i.e. the way that organisational politics is not restricted to management–worker relations but also includes manager–manager relations) requires a revision of the nature of managerial work in the following domains. First, the rational, neutral, goal-directed paradigms of classical management theory and the social facilitators depicted in human relations theory, come to be seen as having more to do with the rhetoric of management than with the practice of management. Second, managers are invariably partisan players in the political processes which arise from and give shape to the structuring of 'organisational' relationships. The position and standing of a manager in these processes depends on his/her reputed and demonstrated ability to shape and maintain systems of order to which significant groupings can subscribe. The activities in which managers engage, such as mobilising, co-opting, mediating, networking, brokering, structuring and contesting, are not neutral in content or intent. Rather these activities are oriented towards shaping and/or sustaining existing systems of order and sustaining the manager's own position within and external to an organisation.[5]

Mintzberg's ten-year study into the day-to-day activities of managers was published in parts between 1967 and 1973.[2] This and related studies showed that managers typically spend the majority of their time talking directly to people, not thinking, writing, analysing or deciding; most of managers' time is spent working in groups, and the largest share of activities regarded as important by managers are those accomplished in groups; managers spend a substantially larger share of their time interacting with subordinates and peers than with superiors; the working day of managers is composed of brief, highly fragmented encounters, most of which are not planned in advance; managers actively seek current, specific, well-defined and non-routine problems, rather than broad, amorphous, or routine ones; managers rely more heavily on orally communicated information, carrying a high degree of uncertainty, rather than on written information, with a higher degree of certainty, conveyed through established reporting procedures; managers use a variety of different channels of information, never relying solely on formal channels. Mintzberg notes that managers in the sample group had initiated only 32 per cent of their verbal contacts and a small proportion of their mail contact. More particularly, it would appear that the bulk of a manager's time was spent 'answering requests in the mail, returning telephone calls, attending meetings initiated by others, yielding to subordinates' requests for time, reacting to crises'.[6] However, as pointed out by Mintzberg, the fact that managers may not initiate contact should not imply that they are playing primarily to other people's scripts or marching to other people's orders. Analysis has to move beyond what is immediately observable (e.g. who contacted whom) and be focused on the meanings that are contained, reaffirmed, propagated or challenged in individual communications. In Mintzberg's terms, a manager shapes the content of communications by:

> [defining] many of his [sic] own long-term commitments, by developing appropriate information channels which later feed him information, by initiating projects which later demand his time, by joining committees or outside boards which provide contacts in return for his services. The manager can exploit speeches; he can impose his values on his organization when his authorization is requested; he can motivate his subordinates whenever he interacts with them; he can use the crisis situation as an opportunity to innovate.[7]

Mintzberg goes on to suggest that whilst many managers 'appear to be puppets', the successful managers will be those who 'decide who will pull the strings and how and ... then take advantage of each move that they are forced to make'. 'Deciding' here encompasses activities on a number of fronts, amongst the most important of which is a manager's involvement and effectiveness in setting agendas. This entails framing the meanings towards which action will be oriented, and framing, invoking and reinforcing rules that will be enacted in particular settings. In *Managers not MBAs: A Hard Look at the Soft Practice of Managing and Management Development*,[8] Mintzberg notes that traditional Master of Business Administration programmes focus on the functions of management. What that really means is that students learn about marketing, finance, operations, etc. However, they falsely believe that they've been trained as managers. The disconnect between managerial training and real-world practice is more glaring in the health sector, where management is shared among clinical and career managers, and life-long learning of technical aspects of health and management training are prerequisites for achieving successful organisational outcomes.

Management interpreted

Managerial activity involves the construction and maintenance of frameworks of meaning and belief systems to which the players can, however loosely, subscribe; and the establishment and maintenance of routines through which particular frameworks of meaning come to be institutionalised and taken as given. The framing, invocation and enactment of meanings and rules usually does not take place in dramatic and obvious ways. Framing as a process is most effective when it is infused in the mundane of everyday encounters, e.g. Mintzberg's ceremonial speech, the request for authorisation and the chance meeting between a subordinate and a superior. Other opportunities for framing meanings and rules are afforded by institutionalised routines, procedures and practices such as the committee 'structure' and other organisational routines such as financial, reporting and employee time-keeping procedures. Henri Fayol, one of the leading 'Scientific Managers' of the early twentieth century proposed four core functions of management as planning, organising, coordinating and controlling.[7] The fact is that these four words, which have dominated management vocabulary since the French industrialist Henri Fayol first introduced them in 1916, tell us little about what managers actually do. At best, they indicate some vague objectives managers have when they work.

Braybrooke[9] argued that accounts of management which consist of lists of tasks that ought to be performed do little to enhance our understanding of management other than indicate 'what we need to explain'. Explanation here requires analysis to be focused on two puzzles: first, whether planning, organising, coordinating, controlling, are constituted by managers as separate and clearly distinguishable activities or whether, as sub-texts in the processes being referred to, they are infused in all of the activities in which a manager engages; and, second, what it is that managers are doing when they say they are planning, or organising, or coordinating, or directing? What is significant about the day-to-day encounters of managers is the opportunities for structuring that these afford them. As managers engage in structuring, they are not likely to make (nor will they necessarily be aware of) the fine distinctions that are assumed when we label some activities as being about, say, 'planning', and others about 'organising' or 'coordinating'. This is not to suggest that particular sorts of encounters, e.g. formal meetings, will not be labelled as being primarily concerned with, say, planning or coordination. However, the labels 'planning' and 'coordination' should not be taken at face value. For example, the fact that a meeting is called a 'planning meeting' does not necessarily mean that 'planning' as set out in the textbooks is the core business of such a meeting, or that such a meeting will be clearly distinguishable from meetings labelled as 'coordination', 'organising' or 'controlling'.

In relation to what managers actually do when they state that they are planning, coordinating or controlling, Hales[10] showed, based on a review of several management surveys, that most managers' activities are best described as: figurehead, liaison, disseminator, disturbance handler, troubleshooting, briefing, servicing, stabilising, monitoring, maintenance. It is the relational and hence, the social and political dimensions of managerial work which are seen as being significant. Management is not simply composed of authoritatively sourced, neutral, technical tasks. A manager's work is social and is constituted in social interchange, mainly through communication in day-to-day encounters in organisational settings. The form and content of what Mintzberg classed as 'communication' are not immune from the settings in which they are occurring. Thus, what is termed 'communication' may include clarifying, obtaining mutual agreement, sharing knowledge, mediating, raising awareness, negotiating, bargaining, networking, reticulating, mobilising, co-opting, underwriting and reaffirming dominant or preferred frameworks of meaning, drawing attention selectively, suppressing, mystifying and creating ambiguity.

Managers who succeed in propagating, underwriting and reinforcing frameworks of meaning which are consonant with their view of the organisation are able to exercise substantial control over how people act and relate, and can do this in relatively unseen ways. To understand how this might occur, it is important to examine how managers use language, symbols, rituals and myth as media for shaping the meanings towards which action will be oriented and thus shaping how relations will be structured in particular settings. The structuring of relations within organisations is rarely achieved by direct imposition, by force or the exercise of 'naked power'. Rather, structuring requires activity on a number of fronts simultaneously. Activity has to be directed at promoting particular frameworks of meaning, values, rules and beliefs and eroding others. The significance of language and meaning as integral aspects of organising becomes apparent when we consider how terms such as 'planning', 'decision making', 'reorganising', 'evaluating' and so on can be construed or interpreted. As implied in Table 5.1, a meeting called a 'planning' meeting can be described as: (i) a meeting in which we will determine strategies to set objectives and coordinate resources; (ii) a gathering to promote participation; (iii) an arena to expose conflicts and realign power; (iv) a ritual to signal responsibility, to produce a symbol (i.e. a plan) and negotiate meaning. Examples of diverse meanings of management activities in organisational settings are shown in Table 5.1.

Bolman and Deal[11] posit that the meanings of 'common sense' terms such as 'planning', 'goal setting', 'communication', 'motivating' are not fixed and unproblematic but can be varied and manipulated; they therefore have to be interpreted in the light of the context in which they are used and the effect that their use produces on other players. This perspective contrasts with how scientific management theory and human relations theory provide managers with ways of talking which cast what they are doing and what they require of other people in rational, objective and socially ameliorative terms. These are 'sacred' ways of talking in that they are more concerned with what ought to be going on than with what necessarily is going on – the 'profane'. Furthermore, when managers or other players use them to describe, explain or justify what they and others are doing, they mask what is or can be contested, and obscure the partial and partisan concerns of those involved.

Pieter Degeling, a leading international health management expert, views the management of organisations as entailing the acquisition of skills to distinguish sacred from profane realms. He underscores the importance of an organisation's managers keeping in sight the values embodied

Table 5.1 Frames of meaning of management terms in organisational settings

Process	Frame			
	Structural	Human Resource	Political	Symbolic
Planning	Strategies to set objectives and coordinate resources	Gatherings to promote participation	Arenas to air conflicts and realign power	Ritual to signal responsibility, produce a symbol and negotiate meaning
Decision making	Rational sequence to produce right decision	Open process to produce commitment	Opportunity to gain or exercise power	Ritual to provide comfort and support until decision happens
Reorganising	Realign roles and responsibilities to fit tasks and environment	Maintain a balance between human needs and formal roles	Redistribute power and form new coalitions	Maintain an image of accountability and responsiveness; negotiate new social order
Evaluating	Basis for distributing rewards or penalties to control performance	Basis for helping individuals grow and improve	Opportunity to exercise power	Occasion to play roles in a shared ritual
Approaching conflict	Maintain organisational goals by having authorities resolve conflict	Develop relationships by having individuals confront conflict	Develop power by bargaining, forcing or manipulating others	Develop shared values and use conflict to negotiate meaning
Goal setting	Keep organisation headed in a direction	Keep people involved and communication open	Provide opportunity for individuals or groups to make interests known	Develop symbols and shared values
Communication	Transmit facts and information	Exchange information, needs, feelings	Vehicle for influencing or others	Telling stories
Meeting	Formalised place to make decisions	Informal place to be involved, share feelings	Competitive place to win points	Sacred place to celebrate and transform the culture
Motivating	Monetary rewards	Growth, self-actualisation	Coercion, manipulation, seduction	Symbols, plaques, perks, T-shirts

Source: adapted from reference 11.

in the profane discourse – of efficiency and rational planning – while being able to recognise that much of the real discourse of organisational management is down to earth and cynical (in a word, profane).

Degeling posits that practising managers will readily realise that there are some occasions on which they will talk 'sacredly' and others on which they will engage in 'profane' discussion. Both ways of talking, when used in the appropriate setting, are means of co-opting people to the speaker's concerns and mobilising them to act in ways which are in line with the speaker's interests. Sacred accounts are used on public occasions such as when the CEO addresses the area health or hospital board, a local service organisation, the local press or a group of newly inducted staff. Sacred accounts also tend to be used in relations with subordinates or clients. On each of these occasions, the manager is concerned to project an image of disinterested, neutral rationality, 'due process' and instrumental goal-directed action. Thus sacred accounts of processes such as 'planning', 'decision making' and so on are used by managers to reaffirm instrumental depictions of organisations, to legitimate both the positions that they as managers occupy and the routines and procedures they superintend, and to explain and legitimate the outcomes that flow from organisational processes.

Profane accounts of organising processes such as 'planning', 'decision making', 'evaluating', 'goal setting', tend to be used with more restricted audiences. With this way of talking, the speaker may be attempting to direct attention to the partial and partisan interests of some of the actors involved and to fashion interpretations around which other actors can be mobilised. Profane talk can also be used to engender a 'climate' for discussion in which partisan agendas, which cannot be disclosed publicly, can be talked about and action can be framed and assessed in terms of its effectiveness in the pursuit of partial and partisan interests. Here, publicly espoused high principles can, for the moment, be put aside, bargains can be struck and compromises and accommodations can be fashioned as participants negotiate with one another pragmatically in calculative and 'give-and-take' terms. Profane talk is used in self-selected (and hence restricted) groups, where talk will centre on partial and partisan interests and meanings rather than abstracted and generally held sacred principles. Thus talk 'behind closed doors', when it is profane, is as much about organising as it is about interpreting, since it is directed to shaping agendas and courses of action to which those involved can lend their support in public forums.[12]

The use of sacred and profane talk in different settings demonstrates the interconnections between talking or communicating, the framing of meaning amongst actors, and the organising and structuring of relationships. In the case of sacred accounts, the talk is framed within an instrumental perspective of organisations, i.e. organisation as neutral, purpose driven or goal-directed instrument. This way of talking, both in terms of the language used and the interpretations given, is used by the speaker to project a 'natural' and 'necessary' picture of what is or should be taking place, which masks underlying conflicts and disguises the pursuit of partial and partisan concerns. For instance, when there is conflict within an organisation, this can be interpreted as a breakdown in hierarchy, or by the thought that 'our goals lack clarity'. In this way, the language of the instrumental framework provides a medium for framing meaning in ways which enable the speaker and other people to make sense of what is taking place. They also explain and legitimise what managers and others are required to do. Emphasising hierarchy legitimises the controlling 'function' of management, while clarifying goals ensures that subordinates not only understand but also accept the agenda set by management.

Meaning construction is a product of the languages, rituals and symbols in use and also of the form and standing of these media. The types of language, rituals and symbols that are used in particular settings are not open to direct and immediate manipulation by an individual manager. Some languages will be more generally accepted in an organisation than others and the language/s in use will not readily be displaced. For example, within health care organisations, the medical model can be seen, among other things, as a language which provides people with ways of interpreting (i.e. making sense of) what they are doing, and what is required to go on (i.e. what forms of action are required, rightful and legitimate). In the past, this language contributed to underwriting a service orientation to health care delivery in which cost considerations were given little standing. However, over the last two decades, a protracted attempt to secure a place for the languages of the economist and the accountant in which meanings such as 'managing demand' and 'containing cost' are recognised and given legitimacy became increasingly evident. More recently, these languages have come to be spoken by a wider range of participants within health care organisations. To the extent that the languages of the accountant and the economist are more generally understood and are given higher standing by funding agencies, the meanings they inscribe have become increasingly important in the interpretation of actions and events in health care settings. The processes involved here have been neither simple nor direct; but have rather been marked by conflict and contestation (Figure 5.1).

The appropriate use of language has major implications for effective leadership in health care organisations. The 'good' leader is one who can get his/her subordinate to do something, but this begs the question as to how this is achieved. An explanation might be that the effectiveness of a leader lies in his/her ability to make activity meaningful for those in his/her role set. That indicates that the leader does not change behaviour as such, but gives others a sense of understanding of what they are doing, and the ability to articulate it so that they can communicate the meaning of their behaviour. If, in addition, the leader can put into words the

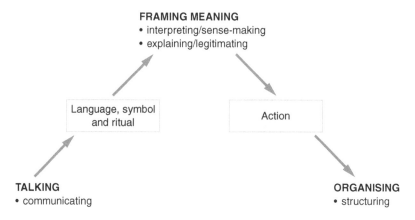

Figure 5.1 Framing meaning in organisational settings.

feelings, sentiments and concerns of the group, then the meaning of what is being done becomes a social fact, i.e. comes to be taken-as-given and not open to immediate challenge. Thus leadership/management consists of at least two capacities: first, to make sense of things, and, second, to express this sense in language which is meaningful to a large number of people. People who have these capacities are able to exercise enormous 'leverage'.

Pfeffer[13] posits that: (1) management is depicted as being primarily concerned with processes such as framing meaning, sense-making, explaining and rationalising, legitimating, routinising, constituting management, shaping and maintaining order without resort to force, and that (2) managers make strategic use of language, ceremony, symbol and setting in carrying out these activities. Proper analysis of management in organisations needs to be focused on the languages that are used by managers as they attempt to structure relations in particular settings (e.g. accounting language, medical language). Furthermore, it is necessary to examine the symbols that are called on, and the frameworks of meaning that managers mobilise in their dealings with other players in the game. By doing this, it may be possible to better interpret how managing as organising, or, in other words, as structuring and contesting, consists of 'sense-making', attributing and framing meaning, and explaining, rationalising and legitimising action. Thus it becomes apparent that management cannot simply be observed, but must also be interpreted.

Doing management

Most formal statements about managerial functions in organisational settings derive from Henri Fayol's *Principles of Scientific Management*, which views the basic functions of management as planning, controlling, organising and leading (Figure 5.2). While useful, this framework is inadequate to fully explain the full range of managerial functions, as discussed in the earlier section. These four aspects comprise the 'sacred' dimensions of the management of organisations. The profane dimensions constitute the other side of the management coin, and require adequate emphasis. In 'doing' management, it is important neither to squeamishly refuse to recognise the profane nor become too entrenched in the 'dirty talk' of 'practical' people that we lose sight of the aspirations of modern organisations to deliver value to stakeholders and address challenges in an effective and accountable way.

Statements about what is entailed in the doing of management have to be based on an understanding of the context in which managers operate. As discussed in the previous section:

- managers are enmeshed in social processes and structures whose make-up (in the constructions of meaning and relations of power and advantage that they embody) are products of action by a wide range of actors (past and present) located within and outside an organisation and hence outside the immediate and direct control of individual managers;
- managers are constantly engaged in analysing and projecting present and future processes and events, aspects of which are continually being contested and much of which cannot readily be apprehended by empirical research;

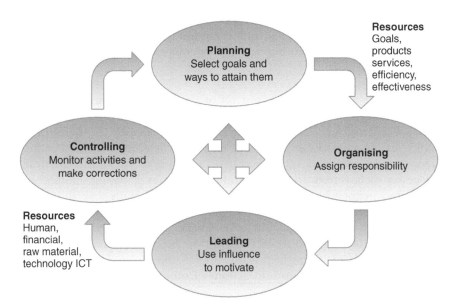

Figure 5.2 Functions of managers.

- managers are continually confronted with social situations in which meaning is ambiguous and contested, in which the outcomes that are produced in action are problematic and in which the establishment and maintenance of order cannot be achieved simply by resort to authority or technique;
- management is a social/political process which, at the level of the individual manager, is concerned with assembling, structuring and contesting relationships such that management entails;
- projecting a sense of order, direction and purpose so as to reduce the level of ambiguity and uncertainty that is experienced by other participants in settings such as a hospital, so that they can understand what they are doing, make sense of what is going on and become committed to particular courses of action;
- blending the disparate conceptions, interests, ambitions and aspirations of individual actors, blunting the demands that are made by contending groups and assembling packages of bargains to which sufficient individuals and groupings can subscribe;
- constructing, maintaining, propagating and/or challenging frameworks of meaning and the rules that are embodied in action within and outside their organisation, with a view to shaping the actions of other participants and the way that they relate;
- shaping, maintaining and/or challenging aspects of the fabric of commitments and understandings which underlies the conduct and structuring of relations in particular settings and, in so doing, influencing how resources are allocated, how rules and procedures are applied and how benefits are allocated;
- mediating contradictions and discontinuities that emerge among actors within and external to their organisation and containing conflict as it arises.

Effective managerial action in pursuit of these concerns has two dimensions, namely, surface and structural dimensions. Proficiency in the surface dimensions of management requires managers to be socially skilled in the various dimensions of everyday encounters. Managers also need political skills with regard to the strategic use of power and facility in processes such as networking, coalition building, reticulating, mobilising, co-opting, negotiating and bargaining, mediating. With respect to the structural dimensions of management, effectiveness is a product of a manager's skill in the strategic use of language, ritual, symbol, myth and drama. Managers who have these skills are able to influence the frameworks of meaning within which actors operate and, in so doing, affect the perceptions, interpretations and actions of other players in diffused and indirect ways.

Management of organisations is, in part, a strategic political process, with managers acting as actors who are seeking to shape the actions of other people. The systems of order which enable power to be exercised in organisations do not exist by definition, nor do they emerge spontaneously. Inevitably, this involves the exercise of power in a variety of ways. In some instances, the exercise of power is obvious and immediately observable, e.g. in situations of open conflict where players mobilise power resources such as control over money, access, staff, and use these strategically to get what they want. However, power is exercised most effectively when it is least noticeable and is seen as being integral to a structuring of relations which are regarded as being natural, necessary and neutral. Where this is accomplished, those in power are able to influence the actions of other players in diffused and indirect ways. As a result, the emergence of conflict is minimised and prevailing agendas of action and relations of power are rarely questioned.

Managers in organisations have interpersonal, informational and decision making roles. As a symbol of legal authority, the manager performs certain ceremonial duties such as signing documents and receiving visitors, and also provides final authorisation for activities on a number of fronts such as policy, resource allocation, performance appraisal, the hiring, firing and promotion of staff. The performance of these surface activities can have structural outcomes in that they can be used to reinforce the notions of organisation as a coherent whole under managerial direction and control. Effective managers know how to exploit the figurehead role in ways which will contribute to shaping people's identity with the organisation, and legitimating the position of management with the organisation. Liaison roles of managers cover a range of activities through which managers develop and maintain internal and external networks and informational contacts with a view to fashioning a predictable, reciprocating system of relationships.

Formal reporting routines provide managers with ways of shaping structural dimensions of organisations. With respect to routine information, managers should recognise that the information available to them from sources such as financial reports will only be as good (in terms of focus, appropriateness and accuracy) as the reporting procedures and routines that the managers have instituted. Thus, it is appropriate for managers to give particular attention to the information systems that are operating within their organisation at any one time and to be actively involved in designing these so that the systems will produce data which are strategically useful. The scope of non-routine information available to managers will be a product of their ability to identify and build relationships with persons who are privy to information not immediately available through routine means but which will be of strategic use to the managers. By combining their role as figurehead and liaison person, managers can ensure that they are brought into contact with a large number of people, and hence can become the information generalist within an organisation who continually scans what is taking place in a wide variety of settings within and external to the organisation. In addition, managers who have positioned themselves at the centre of communication flows are able to expand the information resources available to them by 'trading in information'.[14]

In relation to decision making, entrepreneurial activity is not just about 'having bright ideas'; the successful entrepreneur knows how to translate ideas into appropriate language and into the routines of the organisation. When the latter is achieved, the changes envisaged in the initial 'bright idea' will have been structured into day-to-day life within the organisation. As disturbance handler, the manager takes corrective action on unexpected problems, pressures and changes which are outside the day-to-day routine. She/he is constantly engaged in making short-term adjustments and re-establishing dynamic stability in the conduct of relationships within and outside the organisation. Resource allocation within an organisation is not restricted to 'budget time decisions' but is integral to what a wide range of players are doing on a day-to-day basis as they 'design and deliver a service', make staffing decisions, establish and maintain service networks, comply with industrial awards and so on. When seen in this light, it is apparent that significant aspects of resource allocation are outside a manager's immediate control in that many resources are committed prior to the formulation of the annual budget. This does not mean, however, that a manager cannot, over time, affect the way in which resources are deployed. But to do this, managers must take a long-term perspective, and, in the short term, pay attention to the detail. In the long term, managers have to fashion an alternate 'vision' of the organisation and be skilled in propagating this to other players in a wide variety of ways, e.g. by using and/or altering language, rituals, symbols and routines. In the short term, effective managers exploit their centrality in the conduct of relationships and use their power of authorisation to vet the day-to-day deployment of resources, to fray and erode selected established commitments and understandings, to reinterpret the criteria that are used in resource deployment and, with all of the above, to create 'room for manoeuvre'.

Managerial competence is strongly influenced by managers' skills and technical as well as corporate knowledge of the art and science of management. Most effective managers have a sound knowledge of the history of their organisation and an ability to analyse how the meanings, practices, understandings, commitments and relations of power are embodied in the conduct and structuring of relations within that organisation. They understand how these have been produced over time, are sedimented into various aspects of organisational life and are sustained by relations which go beyond the imputed 'boundaries' of their organisation. An example would be the definition and division of work within an organisation and how this reflects both the history of particular occupational groups, past and present industrial practice, and the specific history of the organisation, i.e. 'the way we do things here'.

Also important is knowledge of a range of social/political skills including the strategic use of power and the expressive use of language, symbol, ritual, myth and drama. Furthermore, effective skills in using these in assembling, maintaining and/or reconstituting relations within and outside the organisation are harnessed by successful managers. Such skills include negotiating and bargaining, networking, co-optation, coalition building, the containment of conflict and the projection of a sense of direction and order. Effective managers are familiar with the languages and associated practices that are being used in the organising (structuring and contesting) of relations within and outside their organisation and their ability to use these strategically. This requires managers to have a working knowledge of the particular language of the accountant, doctor, therapist, nurse, planner, lawyer, personnel officer or economist, to understand how these languages are used (i.e. rhetorically and symbolically) as actors within an organisation attempt to organise their relations with others, and to be skilled in using each of these languages strategically in attempts to challenge or reinforce the structuring of relations produced by the continued use of a particular language.

What has been described in the paragraph above falls essentially into the manager's appreciation of the profane dimensions of organisations. But it should be remembered that in sacred terms, an organisation *is expected* to operate on instrumental lines and therefore it is important that the organisation should be *perceived* to be purposive, that its internal power disposition should be clearly hierarchical and that it should be perceived to be a coherent entity, largely free of conflict. The switching between sacred and the profane, particularly by experienced managerial actors, sometimes leave those who not accustomed to such behaviour with feelings of bemusement, shock or cynicism. However, it should be said that in talking and acting in both the sacred and profane dimensions, experienced managers are simply reflecting the realities of organisational life. If they fail to do so, they would in all likelihood not survive in the organisation, and quite possibly the organisation would not survive either.

Acknowledgement

I thank my PhD supervisor, Emeritus Professor Pieter Degeling, for his substantial input into this chapter.

References

1 Lissark, M.R., Richardson, K.A. *A Management Theory Resource*. New York: Institute for the Study of Coherence and Emergence, 2005. Available from: http://lissack.com/mgmtredef.html (accessed 17 August 2011).
2 Mintzberg, H. *The Nature of Managerial Work*. New York: Harper & Row, 1973.
3 Stewart, R. Managerial behaviour: how research has changed the traditional picture. In *Perspectives on Management*, ed. Earl, M., 82–98. Oxford: Oxford University Press, 1983.

4 Palumbo, D.J. Organization theory and political science. In *Micro-political Theory, Handbook of Political Science*, Vol. 2, eds Greenstein, F.I., Polsby, N.W., 319–389. Reading, MA: Addison-Wesley, 1975, p. 323.

5 Colebatch, H.K., Degeling, P.J. Structure and action as constructs in the practice of public administration. *Australian Journal of Public Administration*, 1984; 43: 320–331.

6 Mintzberg, H. Managerial work: analysis from observation. *Management Science*, October 1971; 19: 97–110.

7 Fayol, H. *General and Industrial Administration.* London: Sir Isaac Pitman & Sons, Ltd, 1949, p. 102.

8 Mintzberg, H. *Managers not MBAs: A Hard Look at the Soft Practice of Managing and Management Development.* San Francisco, CA: Berrett-Koehler Publishers, 2004.

9 Braybrooke, D. The mystery of executive success re-examined. *Administrative Science Quarterly*, 1964; 8: 533–560.

10 Hales, C. What do managers do? A critical review of the evidence. *Journal of Management Studies*, 1986; 23: 88–115.

11 Bolman, L.G., Deal, T.E. *Modern Approaches to Understanding and Managing Organizations.* San Francisco, CA: Jossey-Bass, 1984.

12 Colebatch, H., Degeling, P.J. Talking and doing in the work of administration. *Public Administration and Development*, 1986; 6: 339–356.

13 Pfeffer, J. *Power in Organizations.* Marsfield, MA: Pitman, 1981.

14 Power, J.M. The reticulist function in government: manipulating networks of communication and influence. *Public Administration*, 1973; 32: 21–27.

6 Leadership and health organisations

Leadership concepts

The 2008 World Health Organization (WHO) Health Report highlighted leadership reforms as one of the four strategies of the New Primary Health Care approach. Leadership reforms were described as reforms to make health authorities more reliable and accountable. Health authorities can do a much better job of formulating and implementing Primary Health Care reforms adapted to local contexts.[1] At

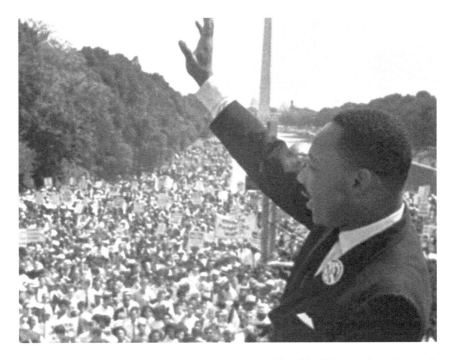

Figure 6.1 Martin Luther King, civil rights leader, giving his 'I have a dream' speech in Washington, DC, 28 August 1963 (source: DrMartinLutherKingJr.com (accessed 1 April 2012)).

government level, leadership reforms in health systems will involve several paradigm shifts. First is a shift from 'reactionary' to 'activist' government, whereby visionary government leaders develop realistic and sustainable change agendas, restrain the pace of change and prevent radical excess. Second, governments need to reinvest in leadership and human resources capacity in the health sector. Such investments should be guided by training needs for health leaders, and the aims of high quality and high coverage of public health programmes. Third, government leaders need to adapt to the rising influence of civil society as a facilitator of health reforms, while ensuring that health technocrats are adequately skilled to navigate the murky but ultimately rewarding pathway of intersectoral collaboration with diverse groups of stakeholders. To paraphrase Warren Bennis, health managers are people who do things right, while health leaders are people who do the right thing. Doing the 'right thing' entails a thorough understanding of core organisational leadership domains (Figure 6.2).

Given that the 'right things' in health (e.g. hospital reforms) are not always popular with stakeholders, leaders need to demonstrate perseverance, be passionate and provide a strong sense of purpose for health system reforms. In relation to passion, Martin Luther King did not say; 'I have a well formulated and politically neutral plan'; he asserted, 'I have a dream' (Figure 6.1).

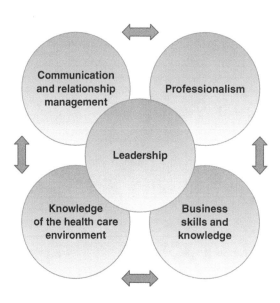

Figure 6.2 Domains of health leadership (adapted from American College of Healthcare Executives' Leadership Competencies site, available from www.nchl.org/static.asp?path=2852,3238 (accessed 1 April 2012)).

The word 'leader' developed from the root meaning of a path, road or course of a ship at sea – it is a 'journey' word. Until the 1940s, the Trait approach to leadership – leadership is innate – in health organisations was popular. From the 1960s to the 1980s, this perspective was displaced by the Style approach to leadership, which viewed leadership effectiveness as being largely determined by the behaviour of individuals in leadership positions. The current dominant perspective of leadership is based on contingency theories, but with the additional factor of leaders requiring vision and charisma to efficiently manage health organisations.[2] The many definitions of leadership reflect its nebulous nature. In the words of John Quincy Adams the sixth President of the United States (1825–1829): 'If your actions inspire others to dream more, learn more, do more and become more, you are a leader.' This succinct quote illustrates the 'functions' of leadership – inspiration, advancement, vision, knowledge generation, increased productivity and self-fulfilment. A useful formal definition of leadership is provided by Richards and Engle: 'Leadership is about articulating visions, embodying values, and creating the environment within which things can be accomplished.'[3]

A remarkable health administrator in the nineteenth century who demonstrated poor appreciation of health leadership was Edwin Chadwick, the major proponent of the Miasma notion of disease causation. Although he was generally successful as a health advocate, he fell short as a public health leader. In the words of Hamlin and Sheard:

> Chadwick's personality was his success and his undoing: he was tenacious in pushing a reform by all available means until action was taken, but he was overbearing and unresponsive to the views of others. He did not negotiate or converse but lectured at people, again and again, until they acted. With no faculty for accommodating differences of opinion, he failed as a practical politician, notwithstanding his ability as a political analyst. After his expulsion from the General Board of Health in 1854 he never again served in public administration.[4]

In contrast, twentieth century British leprologist Professor Robert Cochrane, and contemporary public health theorist and advocate Professor Michael Marmot exemplify excellent health leadership. Cochrane demonstrated the effectiveness of dapsone tablets as leprosy treatment at Carville leprosy centre (United States) in the 1950s, and provided a scientific evidence base to discourage segregation of some leprosy cases. In addition, Cochrane advocated that patients with paucibacillary forms of the disease posed no significant infection risk and should be allowed to leave leprosaria. He was also instrumental in addressing religiously inspired leprosy stigma using medical science and historical analysis of biblical text. In a 1961 leprosy advocacy article, he stated:

To apply, then, the biblical conception of leprosy to the disease we know by this name is unfortunate, for it makes a particular illness, which is frequently a disease of innocent childhood, a religious synonym for sin, and places the sufferer under the mental agony of thinking that he is cursed above all men. The perpetuation of this idea has brought untold misery to men and women, and it is unfair to select a particular disease and suggest that it is a type of sin.[5]

There are many documented leadership styles, some of which may be suitable for different types of health organisations. Autocratic or authoritarian leadership is characterised by individual control over all decisions and little input from stakeholders. An autocratic leader wields considerable power within organisations, and demands that his/her orders are obeyed always. Autocratic leaders typically make choices based on their own ideas and judgments and rarely accept advice from followers. Under an autocratic leadership style, health workers are frequently under increased pressure to provide quality care because task oriented, cost reduction measures are stressed by those leaders who exercise this task oriented style. Edwin Chadwick's leadership style was largely autocratic. This style of leadership is largely incompatible with effective management of modern health organisations, as it alienates potential partners. However, aspects of autocratic leadership have been observed in some military health services and private health businesses such as sole-entrepreneur community pharmacies. Autocratic leadership may be beneficial in some instances in the short term, such as when decisions need to be made quickly without consulting with a large group of people, as in emergency health situations, following natural disasters or military conflicts. Its anti-democratic nature negates its value as a suitable long-term leadership style in health care organisations.

Bureaucratic leadership is characterised by the following: (i) leaders impose strict and systematic discipline on the followers and demand business-like conduct in the workplace; (ii) leaders are empowered via the office they hold – position power; (iii) followers are promoted based on their ability to conform to the rules of the office. This is the most common, and most debated, leadership style in the public health sector. The debate arises, in part, because of the contradiction between leadership, defined as 'the influential increment over and above mechanical compliance with the routine directives of the organization',[6] conflicts with the (Weberian) notion of rational-legal bureaucracy, described as domination through knowledge, and as rule-bound approach to managing organisations.[7] It is often argued that the very nature of health bureaucracies make it very difficult for health workers to be innovative or demonstrate effective leadership. For example, bureaucratisation, which has spawned the move towards increased accountability and community participation, is itself a barrier to effective consultation, because:

Individual bureaucracies tend to respond to a complex internal logic which means their operation is neither transparent to the outsider nor consistent with other bureaucracies. The structural maze of departments which encompass an extremely wide range of programs can appear intimidating, confusing and distant from the community. If the objectives and procedures are unclear, it is difficult for the community to participate constructively in consultations.[8]

Health leaders require rational-legal bureaucratic frameworks to operate effectively, but it need not be a 'machine', Greek temple type bureaucracy which is so regimented that it lacks the capacity to adapt to the changing environments in which health organisations operate.

Max Weber espoused a trait approach to charismatic leadership. He described charisma as 'the gift of grace', and as 'a certain quality of an individual personality', by virtue of which s/he is set apart from ordinary people and treated as endowed with specifically exceptional powers or qualities.[9] More recently, charisma is being re-theorised as theatrical, with charismatic leaders expected to possess outstanding rhetorical ability. Gardner and Alvolio's dramaturgical perspective is that charismatic leadership is an impression management process enacted theatrically in acts of *framing, scripting, staging* and *performing*.[10] Image building is an important component of charismatic leadership. Seized documents from assassinated Al Qaeda leader Osama Bin Laden revealed how much emphasis he placed on image building, from dying his hair to the style of his audio recordings. Charismatic leadership is experiencing a revival in health organisations due to its usefulness in public health advocacy. I define public health advocacy as a process that entails expert mix of five Ps – Precision, Passion, Promptness, Perseverance and Personality – to sidestep or surmount ideological obstacles that impair conditions for healthy living.[11] Passion (i.e. rhetorical ability) and personality (i.e. pre-eminence and image building) are essential attributes of charismatic leaders. However, charismatic leadership has some potentially negative aspects. First, too much passion and too little precision leads to 'spin' and propaganda, which may impair optimal organisation effectiveness by, for example, camouflaging ineffective interventions.[12] Another potential hazard of charismatic leadership in health organisations is that it may usurp rational-legal bureaucratic traditions, and precipitate organisational anarchy. Claiming special knowledge and demanding unquestioning obedience with power and privilege, leadership under this paradigm may shift towards autocratic style if it consists of one individual or a small group of core leaders. As aptly stated in a *Fortune* magazine article of 15 January 1996:

> Charisma is a tricky thing. Jack Kennedy oozed it – but so did Hitler and Charles Manson. Con artists, charlatans, and megalomaniacs can make it their instrument as effectively as the best CEO's entertainers,

and Presidents. Used wisely, it's a blessing; indulged, it can be a curse. Charismatic visionaries lead people ahead – and sometimes astray.

Transformational leadership is characterised by a leader identifying needed change, creating a vision and collective will among employees to guide the change, and executing the change with the commitment of organisational participants. According to James Burns, transformational leadership can be observed when 'leaders and followers make each other to advance to a higher level of moral and motivation'.[13] Bass' Transformational Leadership model was focussed on the extent to which a leader influences followers. He posited that followers go after a leader because of trust, honesty and other qualities, and the stronger these are, the greater loyalty they have for the leader. The leader transforms the followers because he or she has these qualities. Bass' four elements of Transformational Leadership are: (i) individualised consideration – the degree to which the leader acts as a mentor to the follower; (ii) intellectual stimulation – the degree to which the leader encourages creativity and innovation; (iii) inspirational motivation – the degree to which the leader articulates a vision that is appealing and inspiring to followers; (iv) idealised influence – the degree to which the leader provides a role model for high ethical behaviour, instils pride, gains respect and enhances trust.[14] Transformational leadership is a useful style in most modern health organisations. Transactional leadership is more practical in nature because of its emphasis on meeting specific targets or objectives. An effective transactional leader is able to recognise and reward followers' accomplishments in a timely way. This may explain the popularity of transactional leadership styles in modern health organisations.[15] However, transactional leadership styles may stifle innovation if workers are socialised to work towards predetermined criteria. Furthermore, the use of incentives payment may not be sustainable in the longer term, and punishment may discourage innovation.

Leadership is important for both for the organisational process and for consumer satisfaction and outcomes, and higher levels of positive leadership in health organisations are associated with higher levels of organisational commitment, consumer satisfaction and health outcomes.[16] Although there is no single leadership approach that is consistently optimal for health organisations, the transformational leadership approach is the most promising style for facilitating effective organisational capacity building in health systems.

Leadership of health organisations

Unlike business or political organisations, from which most leadership concepts originate, a majority of health leaders are hybrid leaders in the sense that most have both clinical and managerial responsibilities. Health care organisations have complex management structures with diverse professional groupings and professional cultures, making it difficult for a strong and unifying leadership culture to thrive. An important leadership challenge in health organisations is how to achieve unity of vision, given the diversity of, and not infrequent antagonism among, interdependent health professionals. According to Kotter:

> when a high degree of interdependence exists in the workplace, unilateral action is rarely possible. For all decisions of any significance, many people will be in a position to retard, block, or sabotage action because they have some power over the situation ... The greater the diversity, and the greater the interdependence the more differences of power there will be. Because of the interdependence, people will not be able to resolve these differences either by edict or by walking away. As a result, high levels of diversity and interdependence in the workplace are quite naturally linked to conflicting opinions about action and thereby influence attempts to resolve that conflict.[17]

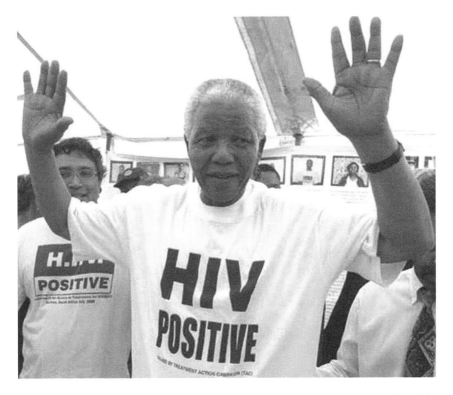

Figure 6.3 Elder statesman and former South African President Nelson Mandela leading an anti-retroviral treatment access campaign in Pretoria, 2002 (source: Treatment Action Campaign, 2002).

This potential encumbrance to effective leadership of health organisations is illustrated by the antagonism of professional-based subcultures in hospital reform. In a study conducted by Degeling *et al.*, nurse managers rejected power disparities that characterise nursing professional's relations with physicians and, related to this, rejected committee-based decision making in favour of rule-based decision processes. In contrast, medical managers preferred a physician-led model of clinical unit management over alternative models that stress management's involvement in establishing work process-control structures and methods (Table 6.1).[18]

Given this operating environment, it is little surprise that the work of hospital chief executives is a high pressure one. In the words of a former British NHS hospital executive: 'all hospitals work on the edge, at the borderline where planning, improvisation and political pressures meet in a framework of financial and physical constraints'.[19] An apparent encumbrance to health leadership in relation to the British NHS government's heavy emphasis on rigid rules is that it had significantly undermined the ability of health leaders to perform optimally. This is best exemplified by the setting of 'targets' – performance indicators which are meant to improve standards, but which in many instances are politically motivated and chosen much for the ease of measurement as for their relevance to organisational purpose. Unfortunately, such encumbrances further fracture working relationships between key health managers, such as career health bureaucrats and clinician-managers, who blame the bureaucrats, rather than the government, for consequent administrative constraints.

In a book entitled *Hospital Revolution*, co-authored by a surgeon-manager Dr John Riddington-Young, career health managers were compared with former German secret police ('Stazi') and blamed for alleged low morale among all hospital workers. The book's authors referred to the NHS management system as a 'cancerous growth' and opined that nine out of ten managers should be sacked.[20] The 2010 government NHS White Paper, 'Equity and excellence: Liberating the NHS', sets out the government's long-term vision for the future of the NHS. This document outlined plans to scrap mandatory nationally determined process targets, an initiative which is yet to be fully actualised due to complex clinical and ethical ramifications.[21]

In the public health sector, professional antagonism between medically qualified and non-medically qualified health workers was most pronounced in the health promotion era of the 1980s and 1990s. This era led to a democratisation of public health leadership and a more egalitarian power sharing arrangement between medically qualified and non-medically qualified public health workers.[22] However, this apparent leadership egalitarianism came at the price of a friction between the practitioners of the science of public health (e.g. biostatisticians, epidemiologists and basic medical scientists) and the art of public health (e.g. frontline health

Table 6.1 Differences between clinical and managerial work perceptions of clinical work organisation

Assessment of	Medical and nurse clinicians	Lay managers
Personalised and hence organisationally opaque systems for establishing the accountability of clinicians	Support	Oppose
Using work process-control structures and methods to address hospital resource issues	Oppose	Support
The importance of clinical autonomy issues versus accountability in management issues	Stress autonomy	Stress accountability
A medical ascendancy model of clinical unit management	Support	Oppose
Using a hierarchical and surveillance model of work processes control for clinical unit management	Oppose	Support
The importance of clinical autonomy issues over information issues	Stress clinical autonomy	Stress information
Stakeholder-inclusive conceptions of who should be involved in setting clinical standards	Oppose	Support
A return to traditional methods for funding and managing hospitals	Support	Oppose

Source: adapted from reference 18.

promotion workers and health advocates). This friction retarded the growth of the public health sector until the Population Health paradigm was developed around 2000 to replace the Health Promotion era. This era also witnessed the increasingly popular name change of the discipline of Public Health to Population Health.[23]

A novel approach to health leadership was developed in 2005 by the United States National Center for Healthcare Leadership. This approach entailed 26 leadership competencies categorised into three domains: Transformation (i.e. visioning, energising and stimulating a change process that coalesces communities, patients and professionals around new models of health care and wellness), Execution (i.e. translating vision and strategy into optimal organisational performance) and People (i.e. creating an organisational climate that values employees from all backgrounds and provides an energising environment for them) (Figure 6.4).[24]

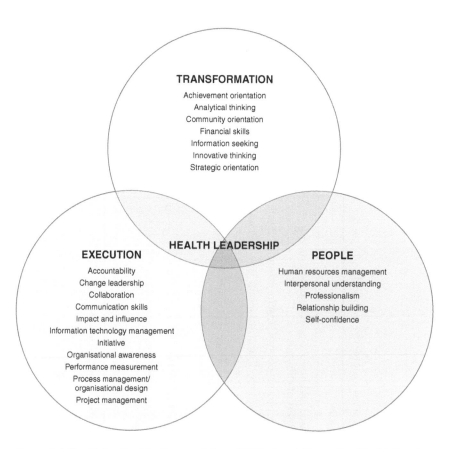

Figure 6.4 Health leadership (adapted from US National Center for Health Leadership's Competency Model (reference 24)).

In conclusion, health leadership is a vital facilitator of organisational capacity building. Leadership is dynamic, in the sense that it emerges, shifts, changes and flows around organisations as leaders and others engage in everyday activities, interpret the meaning and consequences of prior actions and engage in further actions. In health organisations, a collective approach to leadership should be valued, provided a constellation of leaders present three characteristics: specialisation, differentiation and complementarity. Leadership is also contextually situated and practically enacted. This implies a potential for contradictions in the exercise of health leadership in situations of change.[25] Patterson *et al.* suggest that organisational capacity building efforts are more likely to succeed if leaders utilise the following influence strategies in tandem; link to mission and values, invest adequately in skill building, harness peer pressure, create social support, align rewards and ensure accountability, and adapt the environment and capacity building initiatives to facilitate congruency.[26]

References

1 World Health Organization. *World Health Report 2008: Primary Health Care, Now More Than Ever.* Geneva: WHO, 2008.

2 Adair J. *Effective Leadership Masterclass.* London: Macmillan, 1997.

3 Richards, D., Engle, S. After the vision: suggestions to corporate visionaries and vision champions. In *Transforming Leadership*, ed. Adams, J.D., 199–214. Alexandria, VA: Miles River Press, 1986.

4 Hamlin, C., Sheard, S. Revolutions in public health: 1848, and 1998? *British Medical Journal*, 1998; 317: 587–591.

5 Cochrane, R.G. Biblical leprosy: a suggested interpretation. The Christian Graduate, 1961. Available from: www.biblicalstudies.org.uk/article_leprosy_cochrane.html (accessed 15 September 2011).

6 Katz, D., Kahn, R.L. *The Social Psychology of Organizations.* New York: Wiley, 1978.

7 Swedberg, R., Agevall, O. *The Max Weber Dictionary: Key Words and Central Concepts.* Stanford, CA: Stanford University Press, 2005, pp. 18–21.

8 Kweit, R., Kweit, M. *Implementing Citizen Participation in a Bureaucratic Society.* New York: Praeger, 1981, p. 74.

9 Weber, M. *The Theory of Social and Economic Organization.* New York: Free Press, translated by A.M. Henderson and T. Parsons, 1947.

10 Gardner, W.L., Avolio, B.J. The charismatic relationship: a dramaturgical perspective. *Academy of Management Review*, 1998; 23: 32–58.

11 Awofeso, N. Prison health advocacy and its changing boundaries. *International Journal of Prisoner Health*, 2008; 4: 175–183.

12 Linden, A. Identifying spin in health management evaluations. *Journal of Evaluation in Clinical Practice*, 2011, DOI: 10.1111/j.1365–2753.2010.01611.x.

13 Burns, J.M. *Leadership.* New York: Harper and Row, 1978.

14 Bass, B.M. *Leadership and Performance.* New York: Free Press, 1985.

15 Aarons, G.A. Transformational and transactional leadership: association with attitudes toward evidence-based practice. *Psychiatry Services*, 2006; 57: 1162–1169.

16 Corrigan, P.W., Lickey, S.E., Campion, J., Rashid, F. Mental health team leadership and consumers' satisfaction and quality of life. *Psychiatric Services*, 2000; 51: 781–785.

17 Kotter, J.P. *Power in Management.* New York: AMACOM, 1979, pp. 1–18.
18 Degeling, P., Kennedy, K., Hill, M. Mediating the cultural boundaries between medicine, nursing and management: the central challenge in hospital reform. *Health Services Management Research*, 2001; 14: 36–48.
19 Caulkin, S. Crisis management all day, every day. *Management Today*, April 1998: 46.
20 Riddington-Young, J. *The Hospital Revolution: Doctors Reveal the Crisis Engulfing Britain's Health Service.* London: John Blake Publishing, 2008.
21 Sprinks, J. Drive to abolish 'politically motivated' NHS targets raises serious clinical issues. *Nursing Standard*, 2010; 24(49): 14.
22 Rowitz, L. *Public Health Leadership: Putting Knowledge into Practice.* Boston, MA: Jones & Bartlett Publishers, 2009.
23 Kindig, D.A. Understanding population health terminology. *Milbank Quarterly*, 2007; 85: 139–161.
24 National Center for Healthcare Leadership. *Health Leadership Competency Model.* Chicago, IL: NCHL, 2005.
25 Denis, J.L., Langley, A., Rouleau, L. The practice of leadership in the messy world of organizations. *Leadership*, 2010; 6: 67–88.
26 Patterson, K., Grenny, J., Maxfield, D., McMillan, R., Switzler, A. *Influencer: The Power to Change Anything.* New York: McGraw-Hill, 2008.

Part III

Capacity building in health systems

General overview

7 Capacity building in the health sector

Conceptual framework

What is capacity building?

Capacity building is a process for improving the ability of persons, groups, organisations or systems to meet objectives, address stakeholders' needs and, ultimately, perform better.[1] Capacity building is a process rather than a discipline, and generally involves measurable performance objectives, defined outcomes, implementation strategies and outcome/performance measures. The term 'capacity building' originated in the language of

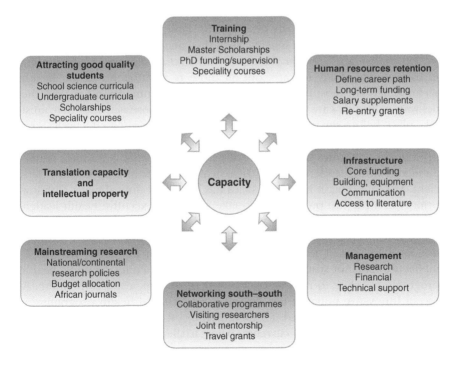

Figure 7.1 Capacity building framework of initiatives to strengthen health research capacity in Africa.

international development during the 1990s, as a broadening of the United Nations Development Programme's (UNDP) 1970s concept of 'institutional building'. The UNDP outlines that capacity building takes place on an individual level, an institutional level and the societal level. In the health systems context, the individual level refers to the individual job performance and behaviours/actions of health workers and leaders. Important elements at this level include: job requirements, skill levels and needs, performance reviews, accountability and career progression, access to information, training/retraining, and professional networking. The organisational level refers to the infrastructure and operations that need to be in place within each organisation to support the collection, verification and use of data for organisational development. Important elements at this level include: management process, communication process, human resource system and personnel structure, financial resources, information infrastructure and organisational motivation. The system level refers to the capacity building functions across different organisations and how they interact, as well as the supportive policy and legal environment. Important elements at this level include: policies, laws and regulatory actions that govern the collection and use of health-related information, resource generation and allocation, systems for management and accountability, and resources, processes and activities across different organisations.[2]

There are several ways to describe the components of organisational capacity building in health systems. First, the concept may be viewed as comprising *strategic* and *operational* components. *Strategic* capacity building refers to institutional ability to carry out all those responsibilities in the health sector which are most frequently accorded to governments, other than the delivery of health care services, and includes all those activities that must take place before service interventions can be implemented effectively. Strategic capacity building focusses on organisational vision and long-term priorities and requires strong policy development, planning, resource generation and strong leadership. In Africa, health leadership is particularly deficient. Most training in health in Africa has been in technical fields, with low priority accorded to preparation to take charge of executive health leadership roles in the public and private sectors. Development of strategic capacity requires long-term investments, which are usually unattractive to most donors, but without which donor programmes are frequently frustrated, ineffective and not sustained. Some donor preference for 'vertical' health programmes relate to reluctance to invest in strategic capacity building. A recent innovative initiative for 'diagonal' financing of health programmes, which addresses donor needs for measurable outcomes, and strategic organisational capacity needs is currently being trialled by the Global Fund for HIV, tuberculosis and malaria.[3]

Operational capacity building relates to activities which make it possible to carry out those activities that result in the delivery of services in health systems. These activities include the clinics, hospitals, private practices, diagnostic laboratories, immunisation programmes and other preventive care services, water supply, sanitation, health education and continuing education programmes. The most common usage of capacity building in health systems is in relation to operational factors, and in particular in relation to training. For example, in a *Lancet* article authored by a former World Health Organization's Information Officer and entitled 'Putting the capacity into capacity building in South Sudan' was essentially focussed on 'training local people to become community health workers in south Sudan'.[4] Capacity building is much more than just formal training. It is not just about improving the people in the organisation but also its other assets. Such assets include networks, culture, financial systems and processes, information management, equipment, infrastructure and governance. Governance straddles both strategic and operational aspects of capacity building. Important capacities for effective governance are shown in Figure 7.2.

Another approach to defining the dimensions of capacity building is provided by the Health Department of New South Wales, Australia. They divided capacity building in health systems into three components; health infrastructure/service development, programme maintenance and sustainability, and problem solving capability of organisations and communities (Figures 7.3 and 7.4).[6]

Another approach to understanding the scope of capacity building is provided by Potter and Brough's 2004 article in the *Health Policy and Planning* journal.[7] They agreed with the WHO description of capacity building extending beyond health professional training:

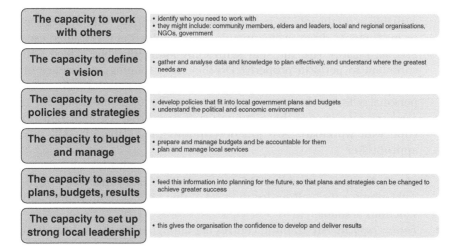

Figure 7.2 Capacities for effective governance of health organisations (adapted from reference 5).

> **1. Health infrastructure or service development**
>
> Capacity to deliver particular programme responses to particular health problems. Usually refers to the establishment of minimum requirements in structures, organisations, skills and resources in the health sector.

> **2. Programme maintenance and sustainability**
>
> Capacity to continue to deliver a particular programme through a network of agencies, in addition to, or instead of, the agency which initiated the programme.

> **3. Problem solving capability of organisations and communities**
>
> The capacity of a more generic kind to identify health issues and develop appropriate mechanisms to address them, either building on the experience with a particular programme or as an activity in its own right.

Figure 7.3 Dimensions of capacity building (adapted from reference 6).

> the creation, expansion or upgrading of a stock of desired qualities and features called capabilities that could be continually drawn upon over time. Capacity building is further defined as concentrating on improving the human and institutional stock rather than merely managing whatever is available … It is unlikely, however, that investment in knowledge in the intellectual sense is all that is required for capacity building.[8]

They introduced the concept of *systemic capacity building*, comprising nine dimensions:

- *Performance capacity.* Are the tools money, equipment, consumables, etc., available to do the job? A doctor, however well trained, without diagnostic instruments, drugs or therapeutic consumables is of very limited use.
- *Personal capacity.* Are the staff sufficiently knowledgeable, skilled and confident to perform properly? Do they need training, experience or motivation? Are they deficient in technical skills, managerial skills, interpersonal skills, gender-sensitivity skills or specific role-related skills?
- *Workload capacity.* Are there enough staff with broad enough skills to cope with workload? Are job descriptions practicable? Is skill mix appropriate?
- *Supervisory capacity.* Are there reporting and monitoring systems in place? Are there clear lines of accountability? Can supervisors physically monitor the staff under them? Are there effective incentives and sanctions available?
- *Facility capacity.* Are training centres big enough, with the right staff in sufficient number? Are clinics and hospitals of a size to cope with the patient workload? Are staff residences sufficiently large? Are there enough offices, workshops and warehouses to support the workload?

- *Support service capacity.* Are there laboratories, training institutions, bio-medical engineering services, supply organisations, building services, administrative staff, laundries, research facilities, quality control services? They may be provided by the private sector, but they are required.
- *Systems capacity.* Do the flows of information, money and managerial decisions function in a timely and effective manner? Can purchases be made without lengthy delays for authorisation? Are proper filing and information systems in use? Are staff transferred without reference to local managers wishes? Can private sector services be contracted as required? Is there good communication with the community? Are there sufficient links with NGOs?
- *Structural capacity.* Are there decision making forums where inter-sectoral discussion may occur and corporate decisions made, records kept and individuals called to account for non-performance?
- *Role capacity.* This applies to individuals, to teams and to structure such as committees. Have they been given the authority and responsibility to make the decisions essential to effective performance, whether regarding schedules, money, staff appointments, etc.?

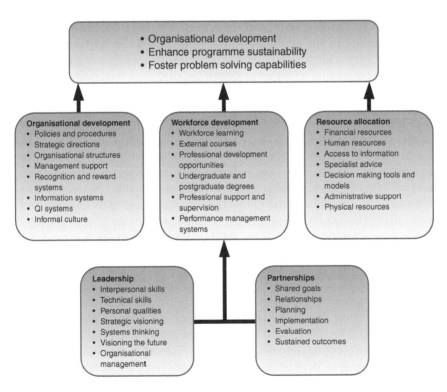

Figure 7.4 Framework for capacity building in the health sector (adapted from reference 6).

Framework for capacity building in the health sector

Capacity building in the health sector is concerned with improving and building the technical and managerial resources within health organisations. Narrowly defined, it is the capacity to deliver specified, high quality services or responses to particular problems. In this context, it is characterised by set criteria of competencies relating to specific skills, procedures and structures, and linked to performance standards, competency assessment and quality improvement. Broadly defined, capacity building describes the ability of a health system to solve new problems and respond to unfamiliar situations. In this regard, it is characterised by diffuse and complex criteria related to innovativeness of public health organisations, leadership, service development, team development and organisational development. The five pillars of capacity building in the health sector are briefly described below.

Organisational development

Organisational development entails optimising organisational management structures, developing management reward and recognition systems, and enhancing quality improvement systems. In 2001, the United States Institute of Medicine developed an organisational development framework for health care delivery, comprising ten general principles; care is based on continuous healing relationships, care is customised according to patient needs and values, the patient is the source of control, knowledge is shared and information flows freely, decision making is evidence based, safety is a system priority, transparency is necessary, needs are anticipated, waste is continuously decreased, and cooperation among clinicians is a priority. These principles are geared towards meeting six specific aims of quality clinical health care delivery; safe, effective, patient centred, timely, efficient and equitable.[9] Following from this report, Quality Improvement Organisations (QIOs), private sector partners charged with monitoring the appropriateness, effectiveness and quality of care provided to Medicare beneficiaries, were established. Examples of QIOs include the Doctor's Office Quality Information Technology initiative (which promotes the adoption of electronic health records) and Surgical Care Improvement Project. The core functions of QIOs are; improving quality of care for beneficiaries, protecting the integrity of the Medicare Trust Fund by ensuring that Medicare pays only for services and goods that are reasonable and necessary and that are provided in the most appropriate setting, and protecting beneficiaries by expeditiously addressing individual complaints, such as beneficiary complaints, provider-based notice appeals and violations of the Emergency Medical Treatment and Labor Act.[10]

Recognition and reward systems are linked to motivation theories of organisational development. The question of motivation is inextricably linked with capacity and needs to be analysed and addressed on all capacity levels: individual, organisation and enabling environment. Potential incentive systems reside within organisations, their structure, rules, human resource management, opportunities, internal benefits, rewards and sanctions. Organisational incentive systems have a significant influence on the performance of individuals and thus the organisation overall (Figure 7.5).

Organisational incentives refer both to the reason for staff to join an organisation, and to the way an organisation rewards and punishes its workers and management. Incentive systems can encourage or discourage employee and work group behaviour. Evidence points to a range of demotivating factors besides pay levels and non-material incentives that can have a significant impact on staff motivation and organisational performance. Understanding what makes people in organisations motivated should also be part and parcel of any capacity assessment exercise. A sensible starting point is to understand and address first and foremost the demotivating factors. Drivers of Change and Power analysis are important tools. Non-material incentives need to be recognised, valued and reinforced.[11]

Workforce development

Workforce development refers to a process initiated within organisations and communities, in response to the identified strategic priorities of the system, to help ensure that salaried and volunteer workers within these systems have the abilities and commitment to contribute to organisational and community goals. Important approaches to workforce planning in

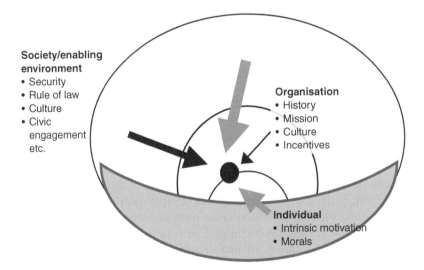

Figure 7.5 Potential entry points for motivation in organisational capacity building (adapted from reference 10).

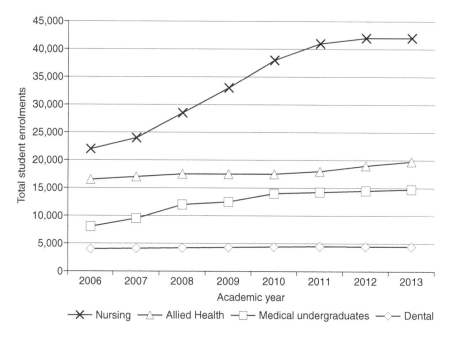

Figure 7.6 Estimated number of students enrolled in health professions in Australia (2010 population: 22 million) (source adapted from reference 12).

health systems relate to securing human resources of adequate quality and quantity, and facilitating their equitable distribution. Greater enrolment of students in health professions is a prerequisite for improving the quantity of health workers. In Australia, for example, the trends in health professions enrolment is shown in Figure 7.6.

Quantity of health workers may also be enhanced through international recruitment of health workers. In Australia, for example, there were about 9,000 overseas-trained doctors in 2009, and this figure is expected to grow at the rate of 3 per cent per annum. This approach to workforce development is highly controversial as it is viewed as a zero-sum game in which source nations lose scarce health staff to developing nations and locally trained health workers face stiff competition for jobs. There is evidence that, within the British Commonwealth of Nations, health professional migration and employment protocols have made a significant contribution to consensus management of the phenomenon, but that it remains a complex and politically fraught issue.[13] Securing appropriate quantity of health workforce also entails striking the right balance in relation to the numbers of various cadres of health workers. In Fiji, for example, the health workforce cadres are shown in Table 7.1.

Table 7.1 Health workforce positions in Fiji

Occupation	Number		
	Filled positions	*Vacancies (%)*	*Positions available*
Physicians	372	24 (61%)	396
Nursing and midwifery personnel	1,957	147 (7.0%)	2,104
Dentist and dental technicians/assistants	171	30 (14.9%)	201
Pharmacists and pharmaceutical technicians/assistants	76	8 (9.5%)	84
Laboratory scientists	–	–	–
Laboratory technicians/assistants	125	9 (6.7%)	134
Radiographers (incl. x-ray technicians)	56	9 (13.8%)	65
Environmental health workers	118	1 (0.8%)	119
Public health workers	–	–	–
Community health workers	–	–	–
Medical assistants	–	–	–
Personal care workers	–	–	–
Other health workers (incl. social welfare, domestic, bio-medical technicians, OT, physio and dieticians)	124	21 (14.5%)	145
Health management workers (executive, IT, administration, finance, etc.)	264	70 (21.0%)	334
Total	3,263	319 (8.9%)	3,582

Source: adapted from reference 14.

The very low priority accorded employment of public health workers despite worsening lifestyle-related diseases in Fiji[15] indicates a poor mix of health workforce, and a poor strategic capacity building approach. For example, the 2010 Fiji Global School Based Student Health Survey revealed that only 33.4 per cent of students were physically active for a total of at least 60 minutes per day. Fiji, with a diabetes prevalence of 9.1 per cent, is ranked among the top 50 nations and territories globally in relation to high diabetes prevalence by the International Diabetes Federation.[15] It is a sad irony that, at a speech on 17 September 2011 to mark the World Physiotherapy Day (published in *Fiji Times Online*, 18 September 2011), Fiji's President, Ratu Epeli Nailatikau, stated that there were four simple ways to beat non-communicable diseases: 'These are to stop smoking, eat healthy food, reduce or stop alcohol consumption and increase physical activity.' Yet, developing public health workforce capacity to achieve these objectives remains unaddressed.

Quality-focussed health workforce development means being clear about the roles of professionals and then ensuring structured training and career pathways that offer the appropriate breadth and depth of knowledge and experience. In Victoria State, Australia, the *Primary Health Workforce Capacity Building Strategy 2009–13* has the following objectives:

> To build the capacity of the state funded primary health sector to plan, implement and manage achievable and sustainable change processes, in order to deliver proactive, person-centred, integrated primary health care; to strengthen the capacity of authorising environments to support organisational and catchment wide practice change and service system reforms; to establish support mechanisms that facilitate the translation of evidence and new skills into practice in order to deliver high quality and co-ordinated services; to increase the competencies of clinicians, project workers and managers to improve evidence based service delivery to people with chronic and complex conditions, and to equip agencies to implement flexible, innovative and proactive processes to adapt and improve systems that support the delivery of person centred care.[16]

Quality of health workforce is assured through strict accreditation of health training schools locally and overseas, and a strong emphasis on continuing education. Changing global demographic and epidemiological profiles also necessitate acquisition of new skills by trained health professionals, as well as those in training, to work effectively in new range of roles in prevention, early detection and management of chronic disease. These include new methods of screening, risk assessment, health promotion and interventions to modify risk.[17]

Developing adequate organisational capacity for improving the distribution of the health workforce is an important facet of human resource management. Currently, over half of the global population is urban based. In some nations, such as the Maldives, economies of scale make the provision of health services to remote islands expensive. Many rural areas lack adequate facilities to make them attractive to skilled health workers. Rural poverty compounds disadvantages in human resources, leading to poor outcomes in a wide range of health services, from vaccination to cancer care.[18,19] Different approaches may be adopted to improve capacity in this area. The use of monetary and non-financial incentives to encourage rural practice, bonding of overseas-recruited staff to work in rural regions for up to ten years, rural postings during medical education, incentives for rural-based students who elect to undertake training in the health professions and improvements in rural infrastructure to make such areas attractive to skilled workers, are among the most common approaches.

Resource allocation

'Resources' includes those things needed to support a programme, such as people, physical space, administrative support, planning tools and financial support. Resources can also include commitment of 'in kind' allocations from inter-organisational groups or partners. Some of the questions that may be considered in deciding whether resources will be made available to support a programme include: will the programme create an ongoing demand for resources beyond the current allocation, and, if so, does this fit with the organisation's goals? If the organisation invests in this programme, what will it de-invest in to free up resources? Will the returns on this investment be short, medium or long term? Who will benefit from this investment? Is there strong organisational commitment to the programme? Are the programme goals and objectives realistic and achievable?[6]

Financial resources constitute a core concern of capacity builders in health systems, as health financing strongly influences the adequacy of other resources. At the government and funding agencies level, arguments over relative importance of curative and preventive health care as well as corresponding funding levels are common. In the United States, the Obama administration announced in September 2011 that it intends to cut $3.5 billion from the federal Prevention and Public Health Fund as part of the President's Plan for Economic Growth and Deficit Reduction. Public health advocates argue that although cutting prevention may seem to save a few dollars in the short run, it will cost an enormous number of lives and money in the long run. In their perspective, preventive health services generally deliver a five-to-one return on investment. Cutting $3.5 billion in prevention would shut the door to as much as $20 billion in potential savings in United States' health care costs in the future.[20]

At the organisational level, an important consideration in optimising resources is waste reduction. In its 2010 World Health Report, on the theme of health systems financing, the WHO stated that between 20 and

40 per cent of all health spending is currently wasted through inefficiency, and that reducing unnecessary expenditure on medicines and using them more appropriately, and improving quality control, could save countries up to 5 per cent of their health expenditure. Other areas for addressing waste include getting the most out of technologies and health services, motivating health workers, improving hospital efficiency, getting care right the first time by reducing medical errors, eliminating waste and corruption, and critically assessing what services are needed, and the optimal cost for service delivery.[21]

Bentley *et al.*[22] have developed a framework for looking at waste in the US health system that may be useful to our examination of resource allocation and waste minimisation (Figure 7.7).

Operational inefficiency is the major contributor to waste in health systems. It refers to the inefficient and unnecessary use of resources in the production and delivery of services. In a population-based study of the quality of Australian health care, investigators reviewed the medical records of 14,179 admissions to 28 hospitals in New South Wales and South Australia in 1995. An adverse event occurred in 16.6 per cent of admissions, resulting in permanent disability in 13.7 per cent of patients and death in 4.9 per cent; at least 50 per cent of adverse events were considered to have been preventable. In the United States, the cost of medical errors was estimated at $77 billion, rivalling the aggregate cost of caring for patients with diabetes.[23]

Leadership

As discussed in Chapter 1, the strong transformational leadership demonstrated by Jimmy Carter was pivotal in the tremendous success of the global Guinea worm eradication programme. In the context of capacity

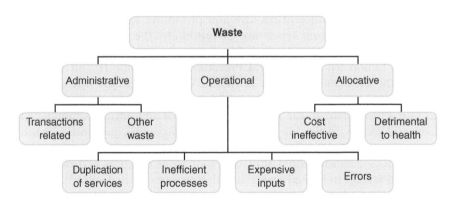

Figure 7.7 Framework for reducing waste in health systems (adapted from reference 22).

building, leaders search out opportunities to change and grow; enable others to act by delegating power appropriately; provide choice, develop competence, assign critical tasks and offer visible support; set example by behaving in ways that are consistent with shared values; engage, mobilise, inspire and collaborate to achieve health outcomes; 'Encourage the Heart' by recognising individual contributions to the success of every project and celebrating team accomplishments regularly.[24]

The inadequacy of health leadership personnel in Africa is illustrated in the 2006 WHO World Health Report. The low health workforce density of 2.3/1,000 population is compounded by the fact that the majority of the 17 per cent management and support staff are not qualified health managers, and most lack adequate leadership training and competencies. Given these deficiencies, who will lead the effort to scale up the health programmes that have been initiated and reasonably well funded in Africa? Additionally, which institutions will be in a position to sustain these efforts over the long term? Unfortunately, building health leadership and management skills are not valued as core priorities by many institutions, foundations, governments or other organisations across Africa. Emerging African health leaders and managers report that stand-alone leadership and management workshops do not provide adequate opportunities to develop a comprehensive set of leadership and management competencies. Traditional leadership training continues to be theoretical and delivered through classroom lectures, rather than through the blend of learning experiences that have proven more effective in helping to develop leaders and managers.

Fortunately, research and practice within emerging successful models in Africa and around the globe are informing thinking and planning for prioritised leadership development programmes and processes, including leadership transition.[25] The urgent need for improving health leadership in Africa is currently receiving significant attention by the World Bank and international donor agencies. For example, the Management Sciences for Health is actively involved with improving health leadership and management globally, but with a strong focus on developing nations.[26]

Partnerships

The development of effective partnerships to address health problems is important because many of the determinants of health are outside the realm of health services. There are two main types of partnerships: strategic partnerships in which systems engage with systems, and local or community partnerships that focus on people. The opportunity to work collaboratively with other organisations (or sectors) is often missed when organisations do not have the capacity to initiate and sustain involvement. The Geneva-based Alliance for Health Policy and Systems Research (AHPSR) illustrates the role of partnerships in capacity building in the health sector. This alliance was established in 2003 to bridge knowledge gaps for enhancing health system performance. Its objectives include facilitating the development of capacity for the generation, dissemination and use of knowledge among researchers, policy makers and other stakeholders. The Global Forum highlighted the need for a shift of attention from 'health research' to 'research for health', which is research undertaken in any discipline or combination of disciplines that seeks to: understand the impact on health of policies, programmes, processes, actions or events originating in any sector – including, but not limited to the health sector itself and encompassing biological, economic, environmental, political, social and other determinants of health; assist in developing interventions that will help prevent or mitigate that impact; contribute to the achievement of health equity and better health for all.[27] Evaluations of AHPSR's activities indicate modest success in supporting research initiatives, in capacity building for health research in several developing countries and in encouraging multiple partners to join in concerted efforts to find solutions for priority health problems.

Partnerships in the health sector may be formalised or operate informally. An example of formal partnership is through a Memorandum of Understanding (MoU). For example, the estimated prevalence of mental disorders among people who are homeless varies, reflecting the area in which the research was conducted, the definition of mental illness and the methodological approach. Despite these limitations there is consistent evidence that people who are homeless have a much higher prevalence of mental illness than the general population. Research evidence also indicates that effective treatment for people with psychosis early in their illness can prevent homelessness.[28] To build capacity to address housing problems of people with mental illness, government health agencies have entered into formal partnerships with government and private housing organisations to coordinate provision of housing facilities to individuals with mental illness. Such MoUs formalise effective working relationships, whereby housing issues can be jointly addressed and monitored at an individual, regional and state-wide level. MoUs also support a collaborative approach towards planning joint programmes, policy development and practice models. Evaluation of various inter-sectoral approaches in responding to the needs of homeless people with a mental illness demonstrates that residential stability is an attainable goal when service systems are well integrated, substance abuse treatment is part of a comprehensive treatment approach and there is a range of housing choices with flexible support available. This then highlights the need for a systemic approach to facilitate greater partnerships between agencies that deliver mental health services, drug and alcohol rehabilitation and housing services.[29]

Capacity building is expected to result in improved problem solving capabilities for organisations. This objective is also referred to as 'learning organisations' or 'quality organisations'. Learning organisations are those which: value individual and organisational learning as a prime means of delivering the organisational mission; involve all its members through continuous reflection in a process of continual review and improvement; structure work in such a way that work tasks are used as opportunities for continuous learning. Changing an organisation into a learning organisation requires a culture change. It is unlikely to take place in a traditional, heavily hierarchical organisation in which the line structure is seen as the only vehicle for communication and control. This impediment to improving the learning organisation qualities of the British NHS was evident as far back as the 1980s, when efforts to facilitate a change in organisational culture – 'the way we do things here' – through a change in strategy summarised in Figure 7.8 was repeatedly frustrated by organisational politics.

Capacity building projects are commonly undertaken with external financial and technical support. To ensure continuation of such projects following cessation of support, it is important to strengthen policy sectors (to facilitate optimal aid management strategies) and operational sectors (to develop long-term equitable professional relationships between stakeholders and training sectors to facilitate optimal workforce development) as part of any capacity building effort. Infrastructure development, a main

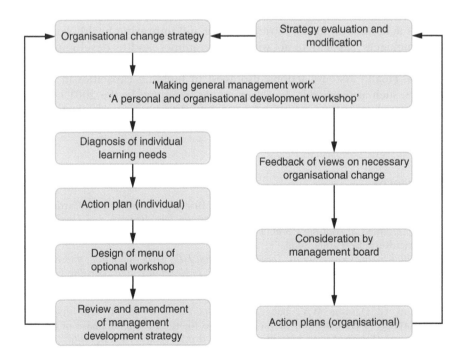

Figure 7.8 NHS's 1986 organisational change strategy (adapted from reference 30).

objective of capacity building in health, has been considered 'economic capacity building' because it increases the capacity of health organisations to service delivery and health outcomes. For example, in developing research capacity, the government of New South Wales has, for over a decade been awarding infrastructure research grants to government and non-government research agencies to:

> strengthen public health and health services research that leads to changes in the health of the population, and health services in NSW. It will direct funds towards research infrastructure support and the provision of an environment in which the capacity to conduct, and use research is enhanced. Infrastructure for research consists of the essential institutional resources underpinning research that are not covered by research grants ... Eligible activities include: Scientific equipment; Purchase of generic consumables such as stationery; Subscriptions to information services and databases; Library resources; Collection, management and purchase of data; Computer equipment and software licenses; Salaries of administrative staff; Salaries of research staff employed to provide general support (i.e., to more than one project), including salary on-costs.[31]

Capacity building is a useful approach to development of sustainable skills, organisational structures, resources and health improvement in health. This is achieved, in part, by strengthening and improving health workers' and managers' capacity to act within programmes, and by developing the capacity of the health system to respond to emerging issues that affect health. Health systems actions also assist in building capacities in other sectors, such as economic development. As reiterated by the 2001 United Nations report on macroeconomics and health, investing in health can pay handsome dividends for economic development and national security.[32]

References

1 Horton, D., Alexaki, A., Bennett-Lartey, S., Brice, K., Campilan, D., Carden, F., *et al. Evaluating Capacity Development: Experiences from Research and Development Organisations around the World.* The Hague: International Service for National Agricultural Research, 2003.

2 United States Government. *Building National HIV/AIDS Monitoring and Evaluation Capacity: A Practical Guide for Planning, Implementing, and Assessing Capacity Building of HIV/AIDS Monitoring and Evaluation Systems.* Washington, DC: Office of the Global AIDS Coordinator, 2007.

3 Ooms, G., Damme, W.V., Baker, B.K., Zeitz, P., Schrecker, T. The 'diagonal' approach to Global Fund financing: a cure for the broader malaise of health systems? *Globalization and Health,* 2008; 4: 6, doi:10.1186/1744-8603-4-6.

4 Bower, H. Putting the capacity into capacity building in South Sudan. *Lancet,* 2000; 356: 661.

5 Reconciliation Australia. Indigenous Governance Toolkit. Available from: www. reconciliation.org.au/governance/your-governing-body-and-leadership/4-3-capacity-building-for-governance (accessed 24 September 2011).

6 New South Wales Health Department. *A Framework for Capacity Building to Improve Health.* Sydney: NSWHEALTH, 2001.

7 Paul S. Capacity building for health sector reform. Discussion Paper No. 5. Geneva: World Health Organization, Forum on Health Sector Reform. Geneva: WHO, 1995.

8 Potter, C., Brough, R. Systemic capacity building: a hierarchy of needs. *Health Policy and Planning*, 2004; 19: 336–345.

9 Institute of Medicine. *Crossing the Quality Chasm: A New Health System for the 21st Century.* Washington, DC: National Academy Press, 2001.

10 Leavitt, M.O. *Improving the Medicare Quality Improvement Organization Program: Response to the Institute of Medicine Study.* Washington, DC: Department of Health and Human Services, 2006.

11 United Nations Development Programme. *Incentive Systems: Incentives, Motivation and Development Performance.* New York: UNDP, 2006.

12 Commonwealth of Australia. *Department of Education, Employment and Workplace Relations Administrative Data.* Canberra: DEEWR, 2010.

13 Morgan, W.J., Sives, A., Appleton, S. Managing the international recruitment of health workers and teachers: do the Commonwealth Agreements provide an answer? *Round Table*, 2005; 94: 225–238.

14 Hall, J., The Human Resources for Health Knowledge Hub team. *Mapping Human Resources for Health Profiles from 15 Pacific Island Countries.* Sydney: UNSW, 2009.

15 International Diabetes Federation. Country rankings, 2010. Available from: www.allcountries.org/ranks/diabetes_prevalence_country_ranks.html (accessed 20 September 2011).

16 Department of Health. *Primary Health Workforce Capacity Building Strategy.* Melbourne: Victoria Health Department, 2009.

17 Harris, M.F., Zwar, N.A., Walker, C.F., Knight, S.M. Strategic approaches to the development of Australia's future primary care workforce. *Medical Journal of Australia*, 2011; 194: S88–S91.

18 Fernandez, R.C., Awofeso, N., Rammohan, A. Determinants of apparent rural–urban differentials in measles vaccination uptake in Indonesia. *Rural and Remote Health*, 2011; 11(online): 1702.

19 Jong, K.E., Vale, P.J., Armstrong, B.K. Rural inequalities in cancer care and outcome. *Medical Journal of Australia*, 2005; 182: 13–14.

20 Prevention Institute. *Proposed Cuts to Prevention Fund are Unacceptable.* Oakland, CA: Prevention Institute, 2011.

21 World Health Organization. *World Health Report 2010: Health Systems Financing.* Geneva: WHO, 2010.

22 Bentley, T., Effros, R., Palar, K., Keeler, E. Waste in the US health care system: a conceptual framework, RAND Corporation. *Milbank Quarterly*, 2008; 86: 629–659.

23 Weingart, S.N., Wilson, R.M., Gibberd, R.W., Harrison, B. Epidemiology of medical error. *British Medical Journal*, 2000; 320: 774–777.

24 Kouzes, J., Posner, B. *The Leadership Challenge.* San Francisco, CA: Jossey-Bass, 1995.

25 Accordia Global Health Foundation. *Building Health Leadership in Africa: A Call to Action.* Washington, DC: Accordia Global Health Foundation, 2009.

26 Management Sciences for Health. *Center for Leadership and Management.* Cambridge, MA: MSH, 2011. Available from: www.msh.org/about-us/technical-centers/center-for-leadership-and-management.cfm (accessed 23 September 2011).

27 Global Forum for Health Research. *Alliance for Health Policy and Systems Research.* Geneva, WHO, 2010.

28 Russell, S., Evans, E. Looking beyond dual diagnosis: young people speak out. Beyondblue research report. Research Matters: Melbourne, 2009.

29 Bhugera, D. *Homelessness and Mental Health.* London: Cambridge University Press, 2007, Ch. 4.

30 Attwood, M., Beer, L. Development of a learning organisation: reflections on a personal and organisational workshop in a district health authority. *Management Learning*, 1988; 19: 201–214.

31 New South Wales Department of Health (Australia). Capacity building infrastructure grants program: 2010–2012 round of applications. North Sydney: NSW Health Department, 2010.

32 World Health Organization. Macroeconomics and health: investing in health for economic development. Report of the Commission on Macroeconomics and Health. Geneva: WHO, 2001.

8 Intervention points for effective capacity building in health systems

Capacity building components: an overview

Capacity building is based on the premise that transformation can only be sustainable when it is initiated, planned and implemented in close collaboration with those who stand to benefit. Building capacity is an objective as well as an approach and a methodology. It provides support to organisations and individuals in reaching their stated objectives. In the health sector, the ultimate goal of capacity building is a sustainable health system Thus, any activity, project or change in environment that improves the ability of a health system to bring about positive health outcomes is considered a capacity building intervention. Building capacity is an ongoing process: there is no final destination. Nor is there a universal standard – a single 'right way' – that all organisations should operate. Each organisation faces different circumstances. An organisation's capacity needs at any particular moment will depend on a wide variety of factors, including the extent of erosion taking place in capacity components. Staff turnover and the failure to update technology systems are common examples of such capacity-eroding forces. In Zimbabwe's health system, for example, brain drain of qualified health staff accelerated following the disputed re-election of President Robert Mugabe in 2008. The erosion of Zimbabwe's health systems' 'structural capacity', coupled with the effect of international sanctions on 'performance capacity'[1] have precipitated major problems in the entire health system, leading to reversals in life expectancy, 3,000 HIV/AIDS-related deaths every week, absolute poverty rate of 80 per cent, ongoing cholera epidemic, public distrust in health systems and acknowledgment in 2008 by Douglas Gwatidzo, chairman of the Zimbabwe Doctors for Human Rights that: 'In recent months we have seen a dramatic deterioration of our health-care system. Virtually everything to do with health is failing to perform at even the minimum expected standards.'[2]

Building Zimbabwe's eroded health systems' capacity will need to take a systems approach, but based on a good understanding of the system components which are most eroded and in urgent need of redress. There are several approaches to examining components of the health system which may be amenable to capacity building in the health sector. Potter and Brough view capacity building as comprising nine facets: performance capacity, personal capacity, workload capacity, supervisory capacity, facility capacity, support service capacity, systems capacity, structural capacity and role capacity.[1] The New South Wales (NSW) Health Department views capacity building as comprising three dimensions: health infrastructure, programme maintenance and problem solving capability.[3] Other capacity building workers take a disease-specific view. This is most commonly illustrated by substantial efforts currently devoted to capacity building for HIV/AIDS management and prevention in developing nations.[4] Controversies surrounding the desirability disease-specific capacity building is closely linked to the broader impasse with regards to desirability of vertical (aiming for disease-specific results) and horizontal (aiming for improved health systems) financing and programme management of diseases in developing nations. Vertical programmes have worked very well for smallpox and Guinea worm control, but have so far failed in TB and HIV control. While the outcomes oriented needs of donor agencies who favour vertical programmes should not be ignored, encouraging all donors to set aside at least 15 per cent of all funding for health systems capacity building is a good start. Using an 'islands of sufficiency in a swamp of insufficiency' metaphor, Ooms *et al.*[5] posit:

> While the vertical approach results in fragile, isolated islands of sufficiency, and while the horizontal approach leads to generalised insufficiency, the diagonal approach aims to build islands with a broad and solid base, and to gradually connect those islands, by helping to fill in the swamp.

Other workers view capacity building components within the health system in terms of funding sources – government, non-government organisations and communities. Capacity building initiatives for non-government organisations (NGOs) is taking on increased prominence in health systems as governments increasingly contract out health services to the not-for-profit sector. For example, the NSW Health Department is currently implementing a five-year plan for partnering with the NGOs to build the capacity of NGOs to enable them to take greater responsibility for delivering family and community services in NSW. Funding is also being provided to facilitate community capacity building. The United Kingdom has invested substantial resources into community capacity building through its Neighbourhood Renewal programmes. Capacity building investments were mainly in the areas of community safety (20 per cent), education (20 per cent), health (15 per cent), unemployment (15 per cent), environment and aesthetics (10 per cent), cross-cutting activity such as administration and community development (20 per cent). The word 'community' has multiple meanings. The United Kingdom Charity Commission defined community capacity building as; 'Developing the capacity and skills of the members of a community in such a way that they are better able to identify and help meet their needs and to participate more fully in society.'[6]

A useful example of community capacity building in the Australian health system is funding provided for consumer participation in health research. This initiative began in 1987 when the Consumer Health Forum was established, and accelerated in 2000, when the National Health and Medical Research Council agreed to fund the Consumer Health Forum's proposal to develop a statement on consumer and community participation in health and medical research, with a premise that consumers and researchers working in partnerships based on understanding, respect and shared commitment are better able to participate in research that will improve the health of humankind.[7] Christine Letts, Bill Ryan and Allen Grossman in their book entitled *High Performance Non-profit Organizations*[8] frame capacity building as comprising three components; programmatic capacity, organisational capacity and adaptive capacity. These aspects of capacity building are discussed in subsequent sections.

Programmatic capacity building

Programmatic capacity building may be described as activities undertaken at four major stages of a health programme's cycle or lifetime, during the identification phase when information on priority health and education concerns in the country are gathered, during policy development and planning to inform national policies and programme design, during programme implementation as well as during the mid to end term evaluations of programmes. Health programme management is a major function of health systems, and the development of capacity for 'situation analysis', 'health policy', 'project quality management', 'surveillance' and 'evaluation' are important for efficient health system functioning.

Situation analysis is a systematic collection and evaluation of past and present economic, political, social and technological data, aimed at identification of internal and external forces that may influence the organisation's performance and choice of strategies and assessment of the organisation's current and future strengths, weaknesses, opportunities and threats. SWOT (strengths–weaknesses–opportunities–threats) analysis is a commonly used tool in capacity building situation analysis. It comprises an internal analysis of an organisation's threats and weaknesses, as well as an external analysis of an organisation's opportunities and threats. In hospital settings, for example, an internal analysis may be focussed on the quality of wound care or level of client satisfaction. External analysis entails, for example, appraisal of government funding priorities in relation to hospital services. For example, a situation analysis of Health Policy and Systems Research (HPSR) in facilitating the attainment of Millennium

Development Goals in the Western Pacific region revealed the following: there is an existing and growing core of HPSR institutions and organisations in the region; HPSR capacity development and knowledge generation and translation are unevenly distributed, with low and lower-middle income countries having weak research capacity and few HPSR outputs that improve health policy and programmes; for many Western Pacific nations, funding for HPSR capacity development and research programmes has been insufficient and short term in nature.[9]

Health policies constitute a framework for framing capacity building actions (Figure 8.1). Policies explain and validate action. Understanding policy means understanding the way in which practitioners use it to shape action. A policy is a projected programme of goals, values and practices. Policies are written administrative or political documents detailing a general and deliberate course of action (or inaction) to guide decisions and achieve rational outcomes. A policy is the formal answer to the question: 'What do we want to do, or not do in our organisation?'[10]

Two main conceptual maps for policy making are *authorised choice* and *structured interaction*. Authorised choice is a top-down approach, with political leaders and 'policy makers' having the responsibility to craft and implement policies. It is formally described as a rational policy making approach, with the nature of the problem, options for addressing problems, how the choice was made and outcomes clearly specified. Structured

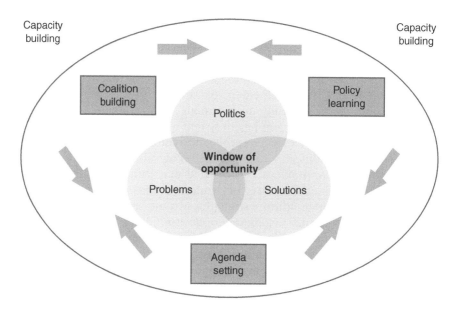

Figure 8.1 Theoretical framework for transforming knowledge into policy actions (adapted from WHO 06.102, available from www.who.int/bulletin/volumes/84/8/06-030593.pdf (accessed 1 April 2012)).

interaction/social construction approaches to policy making focus on the range of participants involved with policy making, diversity of understanding of the issues being addressed and the ways in which they interact with one another to achieve given outcomes. This is a relatively haphazard approach to policy making, but it fits more with the reality of policy making than the structured interaction approach.[11]

Policies play major roles in programmatic capacity building as they provide frameworks for action. For example, Australia operates a Pharmaceutical Benefits Scheme (PBS) which facilitates subsidy of medicines. However, rising pharmaceutical costs necessitate priority setting approaches, which are codified as the National Medicines Policy.[12] 'Rational' criteria for subsidy approval include quality, safety, efficacy and cost-effectiveness. Capacity building for management of rational drug use is facilitated by the appointment of reputable clinicians, health economists, accountants and health administrators at national level to serve on the Pharmaceutical Benefits Advisory Committee.

A Project Quality Management Plan (PQMP) documents the necessary information required to effectively manage project quality from project planning to delivery. It defines a project's quality policies, procedures, criteria for and areas of application, and roles, responsibilities and authorities. PQMP is created during the planning phase of a project. Its intended audience is the project manager, project team, project sponsor and any senior leaders whose support is needed to carry out the plan. Quality Management comprises three process groups: Quality Planning, Quality Assurance and Quality Control. Quality Planning activities entail identifying which quality standards are relevant to the project and how to satisfy them, as well as documenting time frames for quality measurement and metrics reporting. Quality Assurance implies identifying and defining actions, and the metrics to measure them. They provide the confidence that project quality is being met and has been achieved. Quality Planning also includes identifying ways of doing things better, cheaper and/or faster. Quality Control implies identifying monitoring and controlling actions that will be conducted to control quality throughout the project's life, as well as how it will be determined that quality standards comply with, and exceed, defined minimum quality standards.[13]

Surveillance is an important aspect of programmatic capacity building of clinical and public health projects. Population Health Surveillance is defined as the ongoing systematic collection, assembly, analysis and interpretation of population health data, and the communication of the information derived from these data, to stimulate response to emerging health problems, and for use in the planning, implementation and evaluation of health services and programmes.[14] An important component of surveillance capacity is the need to ensure that the Public Health Network has sufficient personnel with skills in epidemiology and surveillance, and that surveillance systems are sustainable and not entirely dependent upon a few key individuals. In Australia, the NSW Public Health Officer Training Program provides a potential mechanism for population health surveillance workforce development. The spans of capacity building for public health surveillance on one hand, and for health surveillance as a programmatic capacity building tool on the other, are wide (Table 8.1).

Evaluation capacity building entails not only developing the expertise needed to undertake robust and useful evaluations; it also involves creating and sustaining a market for that expertise by promoting an organisational culture in which evaluation is a routine part of 'the way we do things around here'. It is commonly understood as an exercise in developing the evaluation skills and knowledge of some, or all, of an organisation's staff, with a view to increasing their ability to undertake high quality evaluations of the organisation's projects and programmes.[16] In relation to HIV/AIDS, evaluation serves to improve the performance of local, national and international surveillance and patient management systems. At a minimum, HIV/AIDS programme evaluation includes the production of timely and quality data on the HIV epidemic, the national HIV response and the use of data for evidence-informed decision making in programme planning, programme improvement and resource allocation.[17]

Organisational capacity building

Organisational capacity building is a system-wide, planned effort to increase organisational performance through purposeful reflection, planning and action. Building organisational capacity typically involves four steps: diagnosing what is missing or needed in the organisation, planning strategies to change the situation, educating personnel to carry out change and evaluating results.[18] Strategic plan development helps organisations both to diagnose what is missing or needed in organisations and how to address such gaps. Strategic initiatives and goals usually result from extensive stakeholder consultations regarding 'where we are' and 'where we want to be in 5–10 years'. Strategic planning is a deliberate set of steps that assesses needs and resources, defines a target audience and a set of goals and objectives, plans and designs coordinated strategies with evidence of success, logically connects these strategies to needs, assets and desired outcomes, and measures and evaluates the process and outcomes. A good strategic plan comprises the following core elements:[19] (1) preparation for planning; (2) vision; (3) SWOT analysis; (4) context; (5) mission; (6) problem statement; (7) strategies; (8) goals; (9) objectives; (10) action plans/activities; (11) evaluation.

Organisational capacity building is closely related to the concept of *learning organisation*. In his influential book entitled *The Fifth Discipline*, Senge defined learning organisations as those 'where people continually expand their capacity to create the results they truly desire, where new and expansive patterns of thinking are nurtured, where collective aspiration is set free, and where people are continually learning how to learn

Table 8.1 Domains of population health surveillance

Population structure and dynamics	Health status	Risks to health	Health systems

A Size and growth
  1 Fertility and mortality
  2 'Momentum' of population growth
B Structure
  1 Sex ratio
  2 Population ageing
  3 Ethnicity
C Spatial distribution and mobility
  1 Urbanisation
  2 Migration
D Family structure
	A Positive health
	  1 Quality of life and well-being
	  2 Growth and development
	  3 Non-morbid processes (e.g. pregnancy, ageing)
	B Health losses
	  1 Disease
	  2 Impairment, disability and handicap
	  3 Death
	C Equity of health status
		A Biological
		  1 Genetic
		  2 Physiological
		  3 Infectious agents
		B Environmental
		  1 Physical environment
		  2 Social and economic environment
		C Behavioural
		  1 Risk behaviours
		  2 Knowledge, attitudes, beliefs, skills
			A Health services
			  1 Accessibility
			  2 Utilisation
			  3 Quality
			  4 Efficiency
			  5 Equity of access
			B Health care resources
			  1 Human
			  2 Technological
			  3 Financial
			C Health policies
			  Including policies in other government department (e.g. Road Transport Authority, Department of School Education)

Source: adapted from reference 15.

together'.[20] Organisational learning involves changes in the people of an organisation as well as changes in organisational structure, operating procedures and culture.[21]

In the health system, it is usually necessary to build the organisational capacity of stakeholders to a level comparable with industry, national and international standards. In this regard, many government agencies are supporting capacity building activities for community-based organisations by providing funding for policy analysts to be employed in these agencies, as well as funding the development of strategic plans. This is one of many examples of health services contracting for which organisational capacity is a prerequisite. For example, the Western Australian AIDS Council was established in 1985. It receives 80 per cent of its total funding from the Western Australian Health Department to provide a full range of HIV-related preventive, health promotion and treatment services. This funding includes a capacity building component which enables the AIDS Council to employ policy analysts and programme evaluators.

In the NGO sector, the following elements are viewed as essential for organisational capacity building framework: aspirations (i.e. an organisation's mission, vision and overarching goals, which collectively articulate its common sense of purpose and direction); strategies (i.e. the coherent set of actions and programmes aimed at fulfilling the organisation's overarching goals); organisational skills (i.e. the sum of the organisation's capabilities, including performance measurement, planning, resource management and external relationship building); human resources (i.e. the collective capabilities, experiences, potential and commitment of the organisation's board, management team, staff and volunteers); systems and infrastructure (i.e. the organisation's planning, decision making, knowledge management and administrative systems, as well as the physical and technological assets that support the organisation); organisational structure (i.e. the combination of governance, organisational design, inter-functional coordination and individual job descriptions that shapes the organisation's legal and management structure); culture (i.e. the connective tissue that binds together the organisation, including shared values and practices, behaviour norms and, most important, the organisation's orientation towards performance)[22] – Figure 8.2. As a component of capacity building concept, organisational capacity building approaches take on a variety of forms depending on the nature of the organisation and its context.

Hamlin *et al.*[23] offer another perspective for organisational capacity building. They characterised it as a staged process, in which capacity building leads to organisational change (Figure 8.3).

Adaptive capacity building

Health care organisations are sometimes used to exemplify complex adaptive systems, described as based on massively entangled relationships, and

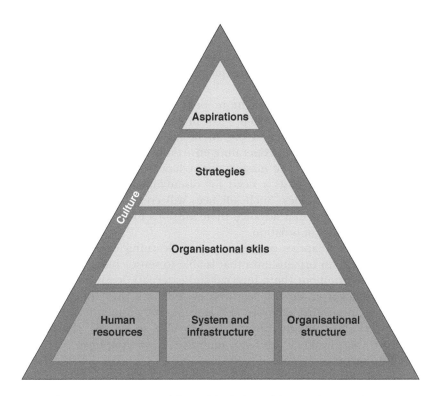

Figure 8.2 Capacity framework for NGOs (adapted from reference 22).

Stage 1: diagnose the present state and identify the required future state

Stage 2: create strategic vision

Stage 3: plan the change strategy

Stage 4: secure ownership, commitment and involvement

Stage 5: project manage the implementation of the change strategy and sustain momentum

Stage 6: stabilise, integrate and consolidate to ensure perpetuation of the change

Figure 8.3 A staged approach to using capacity building to promote organisational change (adapted from reference 23).

having properties of self-organisation, interconnectedness and evolution. Research into complex systems demonstrates that they cannot be understood solely by simple or complicated approaches to evidence, policy, planning and management.[24,25]

Adaptive capacity building is basically the capacity of organisational managers to anticipate, initiate and sustain strategic changes in organisational structures, culture, programmes and vision in order to facilitate the growth and productivity of organisations. Sussman[26] characterised adaptive organisations as having four core qualities:

1   *External focus.* Adaptation is more dependent on the threats and opportunities in the external environment than on the internal strengths and weaknesses of organisations. External focus helps to adapt organisations to the operating environment, and vice versa.
2   *Network connectedness.* The massive entanglement of complex adaptive systems strongly suggests a need for disentanglement, and strategic partnerships with allies. Such alliances will create the potential for system-level effects that advance their missions more effectively than would be possible in isolation.
3   *Inquisitiveness.* Adaptive organisations are learning organisations, in the sense that an organisation that is able to sense changes in signals from its environment (both internal and external), learn from experience and incorporate the learning as feedback into the planning process is inquisitive, adaptive and learning. Organisations that have developed this appetite for inquiry are able to initiate change to improve performance and to embrace it in response to new circumstances.
4   *Innovation.* In the capacity building context, innovation relates to the human, financial and infrastructure capacity of organisations to be visionary in promoting organisational change, and to develop new capacities, products and competencies rapidly. The creation and implementation of new ideas, products, procedures and programmes is an important characteristic of adaptive organisations.

Adaptive capacity building permeates most aspects of programmatic and organisational capacity building. For example, although it is important to define priorities for population health surveillance, adaptations in the form of flexibility and capacity to detect and address emerging and unexpected issues are required for effective health surveillance. In relation to an ongoing (2009–2011) pertussis (whooping cough) epidemic in Western Australia, surveillance records revealed that there were 134 pertussis cases reported in 2007, 468 cases in 2008, 784 in 2009 and 1,416 in 2010. Case investigation revealed that parents and older relatives were among those likely to transmit infection to infants. To address the trend, the Health Department of Western Australia commenced offering free pertussis vaccines for parents and carers of newborn babies. Adaptation implied making use of surveillance data to confirm an outbreak and likely reservoirs of infection, and deploying appropriate resources to vaccinate potential transmitters – carers of newborn babies.

Adaptation of surveillance activities to investigate sharp increases in drug-related morbidity and deaths may provide vital cues into the constituents of such drugs, individuals at most risk, major health effects and their distribution networks. This approach is exemplified by methamphetamine surveillance in the United States, whereby human resources, clinical and laboratory capacity were developed and integrated as part of efforts to control methamphetamine use, morbidity and mortality (Table 8.2).

Capacity building components vary widely depending on ideological orientation, type of organisation, priority issues being addressed, as well as the socioeconomic, cultural and political context. A pragmatic approach is required to address capacity building components, given that some aspects such as 'organisational culture' are not as amenable to change as 'programme design'. Nevertheless, it is important for capacity development efforts to be systematic, and focused on identified components of the capacity building framework. Current evidence suggests that conventional approaches to capacity development premised on planned technocratic interventions fail to grasp the political, social and cultural dimensions of change that are intrinsic to sustainable outcomes. Crisp *et al.*[28] describe four approaches to capacity building in health; top-down, bottom-up, partnerships and community organising. They described the community organising approach as the most ambitious, potentially most sustainable and currently least favoured approach by funding agencies. Each of these approaches has specific components which need to be addressed. When capacity building components are clearly identified, it becomes more practicable to seek funding support, and to evaluate intervention efforts.

Table 8.2 Health consequences of methamphetamine use

Cardiac effects	*Psychiatric effects*	*Neurologic effects*	*Other physiological effects*
Chest pain	Paranoia	Headache	Skin ulcerations
Tachycardia	Hallucination	Seizures	Dermatological effects
Hypertension	Depression	Stroke	Dental caries
Arrhythmias	Anxiety	Cerebral	Anorexia
Myocardial	Insomnia	vasculitis	Pulmonary
infarction	Suicidality	Hyperkinetic	hypertension
Coronary artery	Aggression	movements	Pulmonary oedema
disease	Poor quality of life	Neurocognitive	Hyperthermia
Cardiomyopathy		impairment	Foetal growth
			restriction
			Hepatitis C and HIV

Source: adapted from reference 27.

References

1 Potter, C., Brough, R. Systemic capacity building: a hierarchy of needs. *Health Policy and Planning*, 2004; 19: 336–345.
2 Meldrum, A. Zimbabwe's health-care system struggles on. *Lancet*, 2008; 371: 1059–1060.
3 New South Wales Health Department. *A Framework for Capacity Building to Improve Health.* Sydney: NSWHEALTH, 2001.
4 Taveras, S., Duncan, T., Gentry, D., Gilliam, A., Kimbrough, I., Minaya, J. The evolution of the CDC HIV prevention capacity-building assistance initiative. *Journal of Public Health Management and Practice*, 2007; 13: S8–S15.
5 Ooms, G., Damme, W.V., Baker, B.K., Zeitz, P., Schrecker, T. The 'diagonal' approach to Global Fund financing: a cure for the broader malaise of health systems? *Globalization and Health*, 2008; 4: 6.
6 Charity Commission. *The Promotion of Community Capacity-building.* Taunton: Charity Commission, 2000.
7 Consumer Health Forum of Australia. Summary statement on consumer and community participation in health and medical research. Canberra, NHMRC, 2001.
8 Letts, C., Ryan, B., Grossman, A. *High Performance Non-profit Organizations: Managing Upstream for Greater Impact.* New York: John Wiley & Sons, Inc., 1999.
9 Lansang, M.A., Alejandria, M., Banzon, E., Castillo-Carandang, N., Juban, N. *A Rapid Situation Analysis of Health Policy and Systems Research in the Western Pacific Region.* Manila, Philippines: University of the Philippines, 2006.
10 Lasswell, H.D., Kaplan, A. *Power and Society.* New Haven, CT: Yale University Press, 1950, p. 71.
11 Colebatch, H. *Beyond the Policy Cycle: The Policy Process in Australia.* Sydney: Allen & Unwin, 2006.
12 Australia Department of Health and Ageing. *National Medicines Policy.* Canberra: Commonwealth of Australia, 2000.
13 Centers for Disease Control. *Quality Management Plan Template.* Atlanta, GA: CDC, 2009.
14 Thacker, S.B., Berkelman, R.L. Public health surveillance in the United States. *Epidemiology Reviews*, 1988; 10: 164–190.
15 Jorm, L., Puech, M. Strategy for population health surveillance in New South Wales. *New South Wales Public Health Bulletin*, 1998; 9: 31–32.
16 Beere, D. Evaluation capacity-building: a tale of value-adding. *Evaluation Journal of Australasia*, 2005; 5: 41–47.
17 UNAIDS. *Guidance on Capacity Building for HIV Monitoring and Evaluation.* Geneva: UNAIDS, 2008.
18 North Queensland Executive Training. *Organisational Capacity Building.* Kirwan: NQET, 2011.
19 Prevention by Design. *Strategic Planning Tip Sheet.* Berkeley, CA: University of California, 2006. Available from http://socrates.berkeley.edu/~pbd/pdfs/Strategic_Planning.pdf (accessed 1 April 2012).
20 Senge, P.M. *The Fifth Discipline: The Art and Practice of the Learning Organisation.* Sydney: Random House Australia, 1992.
21 Johnson, R.J. Toward a theoretical model of evaluation utilization. *Evaluation of Program Planning*, 1998; 21: 93–110.
22 Venture Philanthropy Partners. *Effective Capacity Building in Non-profit Organizations.* Roston: VPP, 2001.
23 Hamlin, B., Ash, J., Essex, K. (eds). *Organizational Change and Development: A Reflective Guide for Managers, Trainers, and Developers.* Harlow: Pearson Education, 2001.

24 Zimmerman, B., Lindberg, C., Plsek, P. *Edgeware: Insights from Complexity Science for Health Care Leaders.* Irving, TX: VHA, 1998.

25 Open University. *Managing Complexity: A Systems Approach.* Milton Keynes: OUP, 2010.

26 Sussman, C. *Building Adaptive Capacity: The Quest for Improved Organizational Performance.* Auburndale, MA: Sussman Associates, 2004.

27 Gonzales, R., Mooney, L., Rawson, R.A. The methamphetamine problem in the United States. *Annual Review of Public Health*, 2010; 31: 385–398.

28 Crisp, B.R., Swerissen, H., Ducket, S.J. Four approaches to capacity building in health: consequences for measurement and accountability. *Health Promotion International*, 2000; 15: 99–107.

Part V

Capacity building in health system contexts

9 Capacity building for communicable diseases control

Scope of communicable diseases

Communicable (or infectious) diseases comprise clinically evident illness (i.e. characteristic medical signs and/or symptoms of disease) resulting from the introduction, presence and growth of pathogenic biological agents in an individual host organism. In certain cases, infectious diseases may be asymptomatic for much or their entire course. Infectious pathogens include some viruses, bacteria, fungi, protozoa, multicellular parasites and aberrant proteins known as prions. The term 'infectivity' describes the ability of an organism to enter, survive and multiply in the host, while the infectiousness of a disease indicates the comparative ease with which the disease is transmitted to other hosts. An infection is not synonymous with an infectious disease, as some infections do not cause illness in a host (Figure 9.1).

Common bacterial infections include those caused by Streptococcus, Staphylococcus, and E. coli. The vast majority of bacteria do not cause

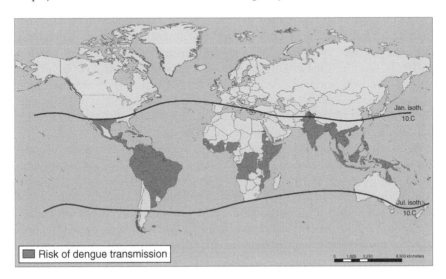

Figure 9.1 Countries/areas at risk of dengue transmission (source: WHO, 2006).

disease, and many bacteria, including *Lactobacillus reuteri* are actually helpful and even necessary for good intestinal health.[1] Pneumococcal disease is a leading cause of serious illness in children and adults throughout the world. The disease is caused by a common bacterium, *Streptococcus pneumoniae*, which can attack different parts of the body. When pneumococcal bacteria invade the lungs, they cause the most common form of community-acquired bacterial pneumonia; when bacteria invade the bloodstream, they cause bacteraemia; and when they invade the covering of the brain, they cause meningitis. Pneumococci may also cause otitis media (middle ear infection) and sinusitis. Currently there are more than 90 known pneumococcal types; the ten most common types account for approximately 60 per cent of invasive pneumococcal disease worldwide. The bacteria often live harmlessly in the throat of healthy people.

Symptoms of pneumococcal disease depend on the site of infection and the age of the person. Pneumonia can cause shortness of breath, fever, lack of energy, loss of appetite, headache, chest pain and cough. *S. pneumoniae* is the most common cause of pneumonia worldwide, causing approximately 35 per cent of all childhood pneumonias.[2] Otitis media can cause crying, tugging at the ear, fever, irritability, poor hearing and sometimes diarrhoea and vomiting. Especially in socioeconomically depressed communities, severe otitis media usually impairs hearing at the age when speech is developing, potentially compromising educational attainment and linguistic skills. In the worst cases, pneumococcal otitis media can lead to deafness. Meningitis can cause fever, headache, stiff neck, nausea, vomiting and drowsiness. In developed countries, up to 20 per cent of people who contract pneumococcal meningitis die. In the developing world mortality is closer to 50 per cent, even among hospitalised patients.[3]

In 2005, the WHO estimated that pneumococcal disease caused approximately 1.6 million deaths, between 700,000 and one million of which were children under five years of age. Millennium Development Goal 4 (MDG4) sets the challenging target of reducing mortality by two-thirds among children under five years of age by 2015. Infectious diseases such as pneumococcus are responsible for millions of deaths worldwide and claim the lives of more than five million children under five each year, making their prevention key to meeting MDG4.[2]

Viral causes of disease include rotavirus and measles infections. Rotavirus was identified as an emerging infectious disease in 1973. It causes one-third (range 29–46 per cent) of all childhood diarrhoea hospitalisations. Application of this proportion to World Health Organization estimates of diarrhoea-related childhood deaths gave an estimated 611,000 (range 454,000–705,000) rotavirus-related deaths.[4] Measles is a viral infection which causes dermatitis, pneumonia, diarrhoea, corneal damage and, in rare instances, encephalitis. In 2008, there were 164,000 measles deaths globally, a decline of up to 70 per cent compared with mortality data for 2000.[5] Fungal infections include Candida and ringworm. Most fungal infections cause mild illnesses among humans. However, they may indicate occurrence of underlying malnutrition, immunosuppression or AIDS.[6]

Malaria is a tropical disease caused by plasmodium protozoan parasites. There are five identified species of this parasite causing human malaria, namely, *Plasmodium vivax*, *P. falciparum*, *P. ovale*, *P. malariae* and *P. knowlesi*. The extent of malaria-endemic countries as at 2009 is shown in Figure 9.1. In 2009, there were 225 million cases of Malaria and 781,000 deaths, at least 97 per cent of which occurred in Africa and Asia.[7]

Hookworm exemplifies multicellular parasites of major public health importance. It is caused by *Necator americanus* and *Ancylostoma duodenale*. It is estimated that around 20 per cent of the world population carries this parasite. Hookworm is not transmitted from person to person. Infected people can contaminate soil for several years if the right conditions are present. Larvae can survive in dirt for several weeks. Infection is transmitted by larvae burrowing through the skin. Hookworm is of particular significance among women of reproductive age, among whom anaemia in pregnancy has major influences on birth outcomes and maternal mortality ratios. Among 251 pregnant women on the Kenyan coast, for example, hookworm may be causing 10 per cent of mild anaemia cases (<110g/L), 30 per cent of moderate anaemia cases (<90g/L) and 17 per cent of severe anaemia cases (<70g/L). The association is greatest in multigravida women, in whom hookworm caused 40 per cent of moderate to severe anaemia, compared with 8 per cent in primigravidae.[8]

A prion is an abnormal, transmissible agent that is able to induce abnormal folding of normal cellular prion proteins in the brain, leading to brain damage and the characteristic signs and symptoms of the disease. Prion diseases or transmissible spongiform encephalopathies (TSEs) are a family of rare progressive neurodegenerative disorders that affect both humans and animals. They are distinguished by long incubation periods, characteristic spongiform changes associated with neuronal loss, and a failure to induce inflammatory response. Kuru is the known prion disease that has caused the most case-fatality. It was common in the Fore islands of Papua New Guinea until the 1980s, and is related to burial practices and possible zoonotic transmission from pigs. Variant Creutzfeldt-Jakob disease (vCJD) is a novel human prion disease caused by infection with the agent of bovine spongiform encephalopathy (BSE). Epidemiological evidence does not suggest that sporadic CJD is transmitted from person to person via blood transfusion. However, there is evidence that vCJD may be transmitted by blood transfusion, a finding which resulted in restrictions to blood donations by individuals resident in the UK in the 1980s.[9] Table 9.1 shows examples of emerging infections and the diseases they cause.

Nearly all of the 15 million people who currently die each year from infectious diseases live in developing countries. In these countries, infectious diseases also disable millions, diminishing their quality of life,

Table 9.1 Emerging microbes and associated diseases

Year	Microbe	Type	Disease
1973	Rotavirus	Virus	Infantile diarrhoea
1977	Ebola virus	Virus	Acute haemorrhagic fever
1977	Legionella pneumophila	Bacterium	Legionnaire's disease
1980	HTLV1	Virus	T-cell lymphoma/leukaemia
1981	Toxin-producing Staphylococcus aureus	Bacterium	Toxic shock syndrome
1982	Escherichia coli O157:H7	Bacterium	Haemorrhagic colitis; haemolytic uremic syndrome
1982	Borrelia burgdorferi	Bacterium	Lyme disease
1983	HIV	Virus	AIDS
1983	Helicobacter pylori	Bacterium	Peptic ulcer disease
1989	Hepatitis C	Virus	Parentally transmitted non-A, non-B liver infection
1992	Vibrio cholerae O139	Bacterium	New strain associated with epidemic cholera
1993	Hantavirus	Virus	Adult respiratory distress syndrome
1994	Cryptosporidium	Protozoa	Enteric disease
1995	Ehrlichiosis	Bacterium	Severe arthritis?
1996	nvCJD	Prion	New variant vCJD
1997	H5N1	Virus	Influenza
1999	Nipah	Virus	Severe encephalitis
2003	Coronavirus	Virus	SARS

Source: adapted from reference 10.

decreasing productivity and creating financial hardships for families.[11] The annual mortality and morbidity due to selected infectious diseases, as at 2004, is shown in Table 9.2.

Controlling communicable diseases

A capacity building approach to communicable diseases control entails first determining the major drivers of communicable disease incidence, prevalence and clinical course, then determining adequacy of programmatic, organisational and adaptive capacity to implement such infectious disease control measures. The following are major drivers of communicable disease spread: population growth and density (often accompanied by peri-urban poverty); urbanisation (changes in social and sexual relations); globalisation of travel and trade (distance and speed); intensified livestock production; live animal food markets (longer, faster supply lines); changes to ecosystems (deforestation, biodiversity loss, etc.); global climate change; biomedical exchange of human tissues (transfusion, transplantation); misuse of antibiotics (humans and domestic animals); increased human susceptibility to infection, due to population ageing; HIV infection; intravenous drug use. Over 50 per cent of the world's population currently live in urban areas, 800 million of whom live in slums. Rapid urbanisation is often associated with the spread of communicable diseases. In England's industrialising cities during the 1840s' industrial revolution, in Frederick Engel's book, entitled *The Condition of the Working Class in England* in 1844, he stated (p. 64):

Table 9.2 Annual mortality and morbidity due to selected infectious diseases

Disease(s)	Deaths	DALYs[a]
Lower respiratory infection	4.2 million	94.5 million
Diarrhoeal disease	2.2 million	72.8 million
HIV/AIDS	1.8 million	58.5 million
Tuberculosis	1.3 million	34.2 million
Malaria	781,000	34.0 million
Measles	164,000	14.8 million
Neglected diseases[b]	173–547,000	18.1–57.1 million
Sexually transmitted infections[c]	128,000	10.4 million
Polio	1,000	34,000
Other infectious diseases[d]	1.9 million	69 million

Source: adapted from reference 11.

Notes
a Disability adjusted life years: the years of healthy life lost due to disability, sickness or premature mortality. Estimates are for 2004.
b Includes: African trypanosomiasis, Chagas disease, schistosomiasis, leishmaniasis, lymphatic filariasis, oncherocerciasis, dengue, ascariasis, trichuriasis and hookworm.
c Excludes HIV/AIDS.
d Includes: pertusis, diptheria, tetanus, meningitis, hepatitis B, hepatitis C, Japanese encephalitis, maternal sepsis and neonatal infections.

As I passed through the dwellings of the mill hands in Irish Town, Ancoats, and Little Ireland, I was only amazed that it is possible to maintain a reasonable state of health in such homes … In one place we found a whole street following the course of a ditch, because in this way deeper cellars could be secured without the cost of digging, cellars not for storing wares or rubbish, but for dwellings for human beings. Not one house of this street escaped the cholera.[12]

Today's slums have not fared much better. In slums of Kolkata, Harare, Dhaka and Lagos, cholera is a common contemporary seasonal occurrence.[13] The spread of the SARS virus between Asia and North America illustrates the role of modern travel facilities such as aeroplanes in the spread of communicable diseases. Intensified livestock production has been linked to the ascendancy of microbial diseases such as E. Coli 0157:H7. When cattle are fed grain, productivity is increased, but fibre-deficient rations can disrupt physiological mechanisms and stimulate propagation of emerging infectious diseases. Biodiversity loss is strongly associated with the spread of vector-borne zoonosis such as rodent-borne haemorrhagic fevers.[14] Other arthropod-borne diseases that may be affected by deforestation and climate change are shown in Table 9.3.

Blood transfusion is a lifesaving procedure with occasional adverse consequences in relation to blood-borne transfusion of disease. Hepatitis C was commonly transmitted in this manner until 1990, when effective screening tests were discovered. Currently most modern health services operate excellent blood screening procedures. However, some communicable diseases such as vCJD remain difficult to screen for, and exclusion of potentially infected individuals from donating blood remain the most viable prevention and control option to date. Hepatitis C has also been spread inadvertently in the course of medical and public health interventions. For example, Egypt's otherwise laudable bilharzia treatment campaign, which ended only a few years before the hepatitis C virus was discovered in 1989, facilitated the spread of hepatitis C through contaminated needles. About one-third of Egyptians aged 50 and older – those who were more likely to have been injected with the tartar emetic shot during the therapy's heyday – tested positive for hepatitis C.[15] In Japan and Canada, Factor VIII vials contaminated with HIV and hepatitis C infected thousands of people with haemophilia who were treated with the serum products.[16]

The theme of the 2011 World Health Day 2011 was 'Antimicrobial resistance: no action today, no cure tomorrow.' Current trends in drug-resistant tuberculosis exemplify how misuse of antibiotics may lead to antibiotic resistance. Drug-resistant tuberculosis is most pronounced in the former Soviet Union, where treatment regimens for tuberculosis are inconsistent and commonly included monotherapy in the 1980s and 1990s.[17]

Table 9.3 Rodent-borne haemorrhagic fevers that are associated with anthropogenically disturbed habitats

Virus	Location	Host	Associated disturbance
Junin virus	Central Argentina	Calomys musculinus*	Mechanised agriculture
Machupo virus	Beni, Bolivia	Calomys sp*	Subsistence agriculture, ranching, deforestation
Guanarito virus	Southwest Venezula	Zygodontomys brevicauda*	Agriculture, ranching, deforestation
Lassa virus	West Africa	Mastomys spp*	Villages with open structures and abundant food
Hantaan virus	Korea	Apodemus agrarius*	Agriculture
Seoul virus	Korea	Rattus norvegicus*	Urban conditions associated with rats
Sin Nombre virus	Southwest USA	Peromyscus maniculatus*	Ranching, construction of highly permeable housing in rural areas
Andes virus	Patagonia	Oligoryzomys longicaudatus	Deforestation, rural construction, monocultures of bamboo
Laguna Negra virus	Paraguay, Bolivia	Calomys laucha*	Deforestation, agriculture
Laguna Negra virus	Santa Cruz, Bolivia	Calomys callosus*	Deforestation, sugar cane monoculture
Arraraquara virus	Distrito Federal and Goias, Brazil	Bolomys lasiurus*	Cutting and burning of native cerrado, planting of forage
Unidentified	Mato Grosso, Brazil	Unidentified	Deforestation, mechanised agriculture, sugar cane monocultures
Choclo virus	Panama	Oligoryzomys fulvescens	Deforestation, agriculture

Source: adapted from reference 14.

Note
* Host distribution wider than virus distribution

The World Health Organization proposed six capacity building interventions to address antimicrobial resistance: commit to nationally financed plan for combating antimicrobial resistance; strengthen surveillance and laboratory capacity; ensure uninterrupted supply of essential drugs; regulate and promote rational use of medicines; enhance infection prevention and control; foster innovations in research and development for new tools.[18]

Increased susceptibility to infection is a common feature of population ageing. Influenza and pneumonia exemplify diseases for which the elderly are high risk groups. People aged 65 and older are at highest risk for complications, hospitalisations and deaths from influenza and pneumonia. Chronic diseases like HIV and cancers suppress the immune system and render affected individuals more prone to infections. In fact, most of the AIDS-defining illnesses are infectious diseases. Illicit drug use increases susceptibility of users to blood-borne viruses like hepatitis C, hepatitis B and HIV. They are also more prone to liver cancer, which further weakens their immune system and makes them susceptible to opportunistic diseases. The infectious disease experiences of the past several decades suggests that health workers and researchers will do better in future in our response to infectious disease risks if they think using a capacity building framework, and act in accordance with ecological processes and principles. Mechanistic 'germ theory' approaches of previous decades are unlikely to be effective in the twenty-first century.

Capacity building for infectious disease control

Programmatic capacity

Developing effective communicable disease control programmes is an important strategy for effective control of communicable diseases. Since the successful eradication of smallpox in 1979, national and international health agencies have shown increased interest in building capacity for tuberculosis control. For example, in 1993, the WHO declared TB a 'global emergency'. Since then, a coordinated approach to develop standard treatments that are effective and promote adherence resulted in the development of the DOTS (Directly Observed Treatment, Short-course) strategy. At a cost of only US$3–7 for every healthy year of life gained, the DOTS strategy has been identified by the World Bank as one of the most cost-effective health strategies available. The strategy combines appropriate diagnosis of TB and registration of each patient detected, followed by standardised multi-drug treatment, with a secure supply of high quality anti-TB drugs for all patients in treatment, individual patient outcome evaluation to ensure cure and cohort evaluation to monitor overall programme performance.

Between 1995 and 2003, more than 17.1 million patients were treated under the DOTS strategy. Worldwide, 182 countries were implementing the DOTS strategy by the end of 2003, and 77 per cent of the world's population was living in regions where DOTS was in place. DOTS programmes reported 1.8 million new TB cases through lab testing in 2003, a case detection rate of 45 per cent, and the average success rate for DOTS treatment was 82 per cent. The 2011 Global Tuberculosis Control Report showed that the number of people who fell ill with TB dropped to 8.8 million in 2010, after peaking at 9 million in 2005. The WHO report found that TB deaths fell to 1.4 million in 2010, after reaching 1.8 million in 2003.[19]

An important facilitator of this significant progress in tuberculosis control is the Stop TB Strategy, a 2006–2015 strategic plan, which aims to enable existing achievements in tuberculosis control to be sustained, effectively addresses the remaining constraints and challenges, and underpin efforts to strengthen health systems, alleviate poverty and advance human rights. The vision, goal, objectives and targets are shown in Table 9.4. It comprises six core priorities (Table 9.5).

The programmatic capacity building approach to tuberculosis control was global and well funded. Such funding included development of national tuberculosis programme action plans which are consistent with the strategy in at least 120 nations to date. Many international aid donors set aside funding specifically for capacity building for tuberculosis control, of which programmatic capacity building was the most funded. For example, the Canadian International Development Agency in 2009 announced a CA\$20 million capacity building for tuberculosis control grant for African and Asian countries, directed at implementing new and innovative or tried-and-tested solutions in TB prevention, care, treatment and support in regions that are currently under-serviced. The grant focuses on building capacity within TB control programmes to address issues including infection control, targeting high risk groups, training lab technicians and health staff, and rehabilitating laboratories.[21]

Organisational capacity building

At the March 2011 Regional HIV Capacity Building Partners Summit in Nairobi, Kenya, many speakers noted that despite a mild increase in capacity building efforts by donors, governments and NGOs in the Eastern and Southern Africa region, the documentation and dissemination of these efforts and their effects on HIV and AIDS programmes and other health programmes and systems remain limited. A reason for such limited achievement was noted; capacity building was very much focused on the objectives, work plans, time frames and measures of sustainability that had been developed by individual projects. In most cases, these projects were donor funded and had their own agenda and hence did not take an organisational-wide approach. There is a growing perception that achieving any desired change that will be sustainable involves more than

Table 9.4 Stop TB strategy – vision, goal, objectives and targets

Vision	A world free of TB
Goal	• To reduce dramatically the global burden of TB by 2015 in line with the Millennium Development Goals and the Stop TB Partnership targets
Objectives	• To achieve universal access to high-quality diagnosis and patient-centred treatment • To reduce the suffering and socioeconomic burden associated with TB • To protect poor and vulnerable populations from TB, TB/HIV and MDR-TB • To support development of new tools and enable their timely and effective use
Targets	• MDG 6, Target 8 – …halted by 2015 and begun to reverse the incidence • Targets linked to the MDGs and endorsed by the Stop TB Partnership: • By 2005, detect at least 70% of new sputum smear-positive TB cases and cure at least 85% of these cases • By 2015, reduce TB prevalence and death rates by 50% relative to 1990 • By 2050, eliminate TB as a public health problem (<1 case per million population)

Source: adapted from reference 20.

strengthening the skills and competencies of individuals within the organisation. What is perhaps more important is the effect of the right policy environment, effective systems and practices, as well as informal practices, beliefs, values and attitudes that must be understood and integrated into organisational capacity building efforts.

Aspirational components of organisational capacity building are important. These components include building consensus on values, vision and mission. Such consensus generally stimulates common purpose among participants. Organisational values define the core concepts or beliefs that underpin acceptable behaviour by employees. In the Western Australia Health Department, for example, their six organisational values are: care, respect, excellence, integrity, teamwork, leadership. Vision describes the over-riding principle that guides the organisation. It defines what stakeholders want the organisation to be. The vision is often the 'dream' (i.e. aspirational image of the future) of the organisation's founders or leaders. Western Australia's Department of Health's current vision is: 'Healthier,

Table 9.5 Components of the Stop TB Strategy, and implementation approaches

1 Pursue high-quality DOTS expansion and enhancement
Political commitment with increased and sustained financing
Case detection through quality-assured bacteriology
Standardised treatment, with supervision and patient support
An effective drug supply and management system
Monitoring and evaluation system, and impact measurement

2 Address TB/HIV, MDR-TB and other challenges
Implement collaborative TB/HIV activities
Prevent and control MDR-TB
Address prisoners, refugees and other high-risk groups and situations

3 Contribute to health system strengthening
Actively participate in efforts to improve system-wide policy, human resources, financing, management, service delivery and information systems
Share innovations that strengthen systems, including the Practical Approach to Lung Health (PAL)
Adapt innovations from other fields

4 Engage all care providers
Public–public and public–private mix (PPM) approaches
International Standards for Tuberculosis Care (ISTC)

5 Empower people with TB, and communities
Advocacy, communication and social mobilisation
Community participation in TB care
Patients' Charter for Tuberculosis Care

6 Enable and promote research
Programme-based operational research
Research to develop new diagnostics, drugs and vaccines

Source: adapted from reference 20.

longer and better quality lives for all Western Australians.' An organisation's mission is its reason for existence. It speaks to the questions: Why does this exist? Whom does it serve? By what means does it serve them? Western Australia's Health Department mission statement is: 'To improve, promote and protect the health of Western Australians by: Caring for individuals and the community; Caring for those who need it most; Making best use of funds and resources; Supporting our team.'

Open communication is an important feature of high performing organisations. Organisational capacity building therefore entails developing an effective and reliable organisational communication infrastructure, clarifying lines of communication and for organisational leaders also need to be actively listening to the ideas, suggestions, as well as the concerns of organisational participants. Capacity building mentoring and coaching of key staff is also important in organisational capacity building. This activity is not synonymous with organisational capacity building, but it is an important component. In South Africa, for example, developing competencies and credential of health promotion workers in South Africa remained problematic due to inadequate tertiary training opportunities for health workers involved with health promotion activities. Consequently, only 20 per cent of health promotion workers had tertiary qualifications. Following a capacity building training programme funded by the Department of Health for 230 health promoters in Gauteng province at the University of Witwatersrand, the several findings emerged: (1) training had provided clarity about the health promotion role and a confidence among workers in being able to describe and 'own' their practice; (2) improvements were reported in relation to behaviour change communication and project planning; (3) capacity building training activities might unintentionally contribute to promoting a sense of frustration among participants who work in organisations that provide little support to innovate and apply newly acquired skills.[22]

Adaptive capacity building

Adaptive capacity for communicable disease control is complicated by the fact that capacity builders are dealing with moving targets, which continually change their genetic make-up and sites of action in order to survive. Influenza virus' antigenic drift and antigenic shifts are classic examples. The rabies virus ensures its propagation by infecting the central nervous system of dogs, thus making them aggressive and vicious. By biting other dogs, these animals are able to propagate. The varicella and herpes virus may remain latent for decades in the peripheral nerves, and get activated when the carrier is immune compromised, thus providing opportunities for transmission. Tuberculosis has many variants, which selectively adapt to facilitate survival in new environments. *Mycobacterium tuberculosis* (human tuberculosis) and *Mycobacterium bovis* (cattle tuberculosis) are genetically related, and *M. bovis* is known to jump the species barrier and infect humans.[23] A 2011 DNA sequencing study of *Yersinia pestis* showed that the common ancestor of the several variants of this plague-causing bacterium emerged around the early thirteenth century.[24] Thus, the double burden of adaptive capacity building in communicable disease control comprises defining and predicting the adaptations of infectious agents on one hand, and reforming health organisations and programmes to cope with such anticipated shifts and drifts in the genes and predilections of infectious agents. Two examples will be used to illustrate adaptive capacity building for infectious diseases – leprosy (a stable chronic bacterial) and influenza (an acute and unstable viral disease).

Leprosy management is a unique example of ongoing adaptive capacity building in the health sector. As at 2009, there were 244,915 registered cases of leprosy globally, a dramatic decrease from 5.2 million cases in 1995. Leprosy is a chronic disease caused by a bacillus, *Mycobacterium leprae*. Leprosy is not highly infectious. It is transmitted via droplets, from the nose and mouth, during close and frequent contacts with untreated cases. Untreated, leprosy can cause progressive and permanent damage to the skin, nerves, limbs and eyes. With the global prevalence of leprosy dropping to below one per 10,000 global inhabitants in 2000, it became necessary to reorganise vertical leprosy services into the general health services in order to take advantages of economies of scale and hopefully reduce stigma. In Orissa leprosy programme, India, this adaptation occurred in two stages – functional integration, and integration of the leprosy programme infrastructure. functional integration included training primary health care (PHC) staff to diagnose and manage leprosy and its complications, to maintain MDT stocks, to record and report cases and carry out information, education and communication activities. Structural integration entailed posting leprosy-trained paramedical workers from the vertical programme into PHC clinics and establishing a district nucleus of four to seven specialised leprosy workers 'nested' in each local government area. Orissa state successfully implemented integration of an elimination programme into its primary health care system. Continuous monitoring of the programme and timely action enabled the programme to adapt quickly to the PHC environment.[25]

Such successful adaptation of leprosy control's organisational structures requires exceptional organisational skills. Visschedijk *et al.*[26] proposed a staged approach comprising situation analysis (strengths, weaknesses, threats and opportunities of integration), analysing weaknesses, strengths and priorities, ensuring commitment to integration by decision makers, developing a plan for the integration process, making adaptation preparations, implementing and monitoring, and evaluating. In the author's experience in implementing leprosy integration programmes, the most problematic organisational issues include training of leprosy workers to work within the PHC system, addressing stigma by health workers and non-leprosy patients, and infrastructural integration, especially of considerable leprosy resources, which may sometimes imply a reverse integration of PHC services into the physical infrastructure of leprosy facilities.[27]

Seasonal influenza is a viral infection that affects mainly the nose, throat, bronchi and, occasionally, lungs. Infection usually lasts for about a week, and is characterised by sudden onset of high fever, aching muscles, headache and severe malaise, non-productive cough, sore throat and rhinitis. The virus is transmitted easily from person to person via droplets and small particles produced when infected people cough or sneeze. Influenza tends to spread rapidly in seasonal epidemics. Most infected people recover within one to two weeks without requiring medical treatment. However, in the very young, the elderly and those with other serious medical conditions, infection can lead to severe complications of the underlying condition, pneumonia and death. There are three types of seasonal influenza – A, B and C. Type A influenza viruses are further typed into subtypes according to different kinds and combinations of virus surface proteins. Among many subtypes of influenza A viruses, currently influenza A(H1N1) and A(H3N2) subtypes are circulating among humans. Influenza viruses circulate in every part of the world. Type C influenza cases occur much less frequently than A and B. That is why only influenza A and B viruses are included in seasonal influenza vaccines.[28] Pandemic influenza describes either a known strain of influenza which has acquired increased virulence, or an exotic strain of influenza, either of which have spread across three WHO regions, and are spread by human-to-human contact. A recent example is the April 2009 H1N1 influenza pandemic, which moved into the post-pandemic phase in August 2010, following 1,549,364 cases and 25,174 deaths (1.62 per cent case fatality rate). H1N1 is considered seasonal influenza in the 2011 vaccine formulation.[29]

Programmatic capacity building for seasonal influenza control is essentially comprised of implementing an influenza vaccination programme, and providing resources for managing increased numbers of patients presenting with influenza-like illness during the influenza season. As the vaccines need to be reformulated every year, and since they provide up to 12 months' protection, individuals at risk of seasonal influenza are encouraged by influenza control programme managers to get vaccinated. This has been a difficult objective given doubts about the efficacy of influenza vaccine even by health workers. For example, in the United States, a September 2011 survey of 1,931 health workers, conducted by the Centers for Disease Control, showed that only 63.5 per cent had received the vaccine for the 2010–2011 season. Adapting to the campaigns of the anti-immunisation lobby involves responding with facts, packaged such that it refutes the arguments of the anti-immunisation lobby, and is extensively disseminated. An example of such document, entitled *Immunisation Myths and Realities: Responding to Arguments against Immunisation,*[30] was produced by Australia's Department of Health, and is currently in its fourth edition as it updates information in response to emerging concerns. At times of low influenza activity such as the 2011–2012 influenza season, there is usually little motivation for individuals to get vaccinated. Influenza control capacity building also entails building adequate clinical capacity to anticipate and manage excess emergency presentations for influenza. Seasonal influenza control programmes entail urging people to take everyday actions to prevent the spread of influenza. These massages aim to appropriately devolve responsibility for flu transmission reduction to community members, as reflected in the following message from the Centers for Disease Control:

> Cover your nose and mouth with a tissue when you cough or sneeze. Throw the tissue in the trash after you use it; Wash your hands often with soap and water. If soap and water are not available, use an alcohol-based hand rub; Avoid touching your eyes, nose and mouth. Germs spread this way; Try to avoid close contact with sick people; If you are sick with flu-like illness, CDC recommends that you stay home for at least 24 hours after your fever is gone except to get medical care or for other necessities. (Your fever should be gone without the use of a fever-reducing medicine.) While sick, limit contact with others as much as possible to keep from infecting them; take flu antiviral drugs if your doctor prescribes them.[31]

Adaptations in capacity building are especially important in developing adequate organisational structures to predict estimates of additional vaccines and presentations to emergency hospitals, and to deploy human resources to influenza control as appropriate. Given the substantial human and financial resources devoted to influenza surveillance, control, treatment and prevention, it is surprising that very little is known about the actual burden of disease proven – not modelled to be due to influenza. After almost a decade of the United States' Centers for Disease Control stating that influenza is estimated to kill 36,000 Americans annually, it revised the figure downward to 24,000 in 2010, and currently states that 4,000 to 40,000 deaths may occur annually due to influenza. Such 'guesswork' estimates of morbidity and mortality for a disease around which at least 250 million doses of vaccines are administered annually indicates poor organisational capacity for influenza control.

Adapting to the regularly changing patterns of influenza viruses requires investments in research to produce vaccines which share core attributes of most influenza vaccines and has longer efficacy than the 12 months' protection offered by current vaccines. Given relatively low influenza prevalence over the past two decades, it may be prudent to consider the cost-effectiveness of current approaches to influenza control. A study undertaken by the author in New South Wales prisons demonstrated that, for outbreaks occurring once every ten years, antiviral medication provision to those infected was more cost-effective than annual influenza vaccination.[32]

Communicable diseases are returning with a vengeance at the beginning of the twenty-first century. Approximately 35 new emerging and re-emerging infectious diseases have been identified as global threats since 1980. Some communicable diseases, such as cholera, malaria, HIV and tuberculosis have common characteristics that facilitate them being controlled collectively and effectively – they are closely related to poverty, social inequities, poor living conditions, risky health behaviours and inefficient health care delivery. Others, such as leprosy and influenza, are more amorphous, and require massive investments in basic research, in addition to major adaptations in current control strategies. Nevertheless, common themes in organisational capacity for communicable disease control are:[10]

- research into cost-effectiveness of infection control strategies should be encouraged:
- government leadership and sustained commitment is critically important;
- active participation by civil society is essential;
- managed decentralisation can be effective;
- human resources development is critical;
- intersectoral policies and programmes need to be strengthened;
- sound information and surveillance systems are urgently needed.

The successes documented with current efforts to achieve Guinea worm eradication over the next five years, discussed in Chapter 1, are largely attributed to enhanced organisational capacity building efforts led by former US President Jimmy Carter. Similar impressive results are possible with most other communicable diseases if careful attention is devoted to programmatic, organisational and adaptive capacity building efforts.

References

1 Miyoshi, A., Rocha, C.S., Azevedo, V., LeBlanc, J.G. Potential application of probiotics in the prevention and treatment of inflammatory bowel diseases. *Ulcers*, 2011; Article ID 841651.
2 The All-Party Parliamentary Group. *Improving Global Health by Preventing Haemophiliac Disease*. New York: GAVI, 2008.
3 Goetghebuer, T., West, T.E., Wermenbol, V., Cadbury, A.L., Milligan, P., Lloyd-Evans, N., *et al.* Outcome of meningitis caused by *Streptococcus pneumonia and Haemophilus influenza* type b in children in the Gambia. *Tropical Medicine and International Health*, 2000; 5: 207–213.
4 Parashar, U.D., Gibson, C.J., Bresee, J.S., Glass, R.I. Rotavirus and severe childhood diarrhoea. *Emerging Infectious Diseases*, 2006; 12: 304–306.
5 World Health Organization. *Measles Factsheet 286, October 2011*. Geneva: WHO, 2011.
6 Moazeni, M., Haghmorad, D., Mirshafiey, A. Opportunistic fungal infections in patients with HIV and AIDS. *Journal of Chinese Clinical Medicine*, 2009; 4: 106–120.

7 World Health Organization. *World Malaria Report, 2010.* Geneva: WHO, 2010.
8 Shulman, C.E., Graham, W.J., Jilo, H., Lowe, B.S., New, L., Obiero, J., *et al.* Malaria is an important cause of anaemia in primigravidae: evidence from a district hospital in coastal Kenya. *Transactions of Royal Society of Tropical Medicine and Hygiene,* 1996; 90: 535–539.
9 Llewelyn, C.A., Hewitt, P.E., Knight, R.S.G. Possible transmission of variant Creutzfeldt-Jakob disease by blood transfusion. *Lancet,* 2004; 363: 417–421.
10 Coker, R., Atun, R., McKee, M. *Health Systems and the Challenge of Communicable Diseases: Experiences from Europe and Latin America.* Maidenhead, England: Open University Press, 2007.
11 Global Health Council. *Mortality and Morbidity of Infectious Diseases, 2004.* Washington, DC: GHC, 2009.
12 Engels, F. *The Condition of the Working-Class in England in 1844.* Translated by Florence Kelley Wischnewetzky from the January 1943 George Allen & Unwin reprint of the March 1892 edition by David Price. Available from: www.gutenberg.org/files/17306/17306-h/17306-h.htm (accessed 1 April 2012).
13 Sur, D., Deen, J., Manna, B., Niyogi, S.K., Deb, A.K., Kanungo, S., *et al.* The burden of cholera in the slums of Kolkata, India: data from a prospective, community based study. *Archives of Diseases of Children,* 2005; 90: 1175–1181.
14 Mills, J.N. Biodiversity loss and emerging infectious disease: an example from the rodent-borne hemorrhagic fevers. *Biodiversity,* 2006; 7: 9–17.
15 Pybus, O.G., Drummond, A.J., Nakano, T., Robertson, B.H., Rambaut, A. The epidemiology and iatrogenic transmission of hepatitis C virus in Egypt: a Bayesian coalescent approach. *Molecular Biology and Evolution,* 2003; 20: 381–387.
16 Dunn, K. HIV and Canada's haemophiliacs: looking back at a tragedy. *Canadian Medical Association Journal,* 1993; 148: 609–612.
17 World Health Organization. *Estimated Number of Multidrug Resistant Tuberculosis Cases, 2009.* Geneva: WHO, 2011.
18 World Health Organization. *World Health Day 2011.* Geneva: WHO, 2011.
19 World Health organization. *2011 Global Tuberculosis Control Report.* Geneva, WHO, 2011.
20 World Health Organisation. *The Stop TB Strategy.* Geneva: WHO, 2006.
21 Canadian International Development Agency. Capacity Building for Tuberculosis Control. Project M012620-001, 23 March 2009.
22 Mills, J., Rudolph, M. Health promotion capacity building in South Africa. *Global Health Promotion,* 2010; 17: 29–34.
23 Park, D., Qin, H., Jain, S. Tuberculosis due to *Mycobacterium bovis* in patients coinfected with human immunodeficiency virus. *Clinical Infectious Diseases,* 2010; 51: 1343–1346. Doi: 10.1086/657118.
24 Bos, K.I., Schuenemann, V.J., Golding, G.B., Burbano, H.A., Waglechner, N., Coombes, B.K., *et al.* A draft genome of *Yersinia pestis* from victims of the Black Death. *Nature,* 2011; 480: 278.
25 Siddiqui, M.R., Velidi, N.R., Pati, S., Rath, N., Kanungo, A.K., Bhanjadeo, A.K., *et al.* Integration of leprosy elimination into primary health care in Orissa, India. *PloS One,* 2009, 4(12): e8351. Doi:10.1371/journal.pone.0008351.
26 Visschedijk, J., Engelhard, A., Lever, P., Grossi, M.A.F., Feenstra, P. Leprosy control strategies and the integration of health services: an international perspective. *Cadernos de Saúde Pública,* 2003; 19: 1567–1581.
27 Awofeso, N. Life after multidrug therapy: the managerial implications in leprosy control in Kaduna State, Nigeria. *Tropical Doctor,* 1997; 27: 196–198.
28 World Health Organization. *Seasonal Influenza Factsheet 211.* Geneva: WHO, 2009.
29 Centers for Disease Control. *Swine Flu Count.* Atlanta, GA: CDC, 2010.

30 Commonwealth of Australia. *Immunisation Myths and Realities: Responding to Arguments against Immunisation – A Guide for Providers.* Canberra: Department of Health and Ageing, 2008.
31 Centers for Disease Control. *'Take 3' Actions to Fight the Flu.* Atlanta, GA: CDC, 2011.
32 Awofeso, N., Rawlinson, W.D. Influenza control in Australian prison settings: cost–benefit analysis of major strategies. *International Journal of Prisoner Health,* 2005; 1: 25–31.

10 Capacity building for non-communicable diseases control

The concept of non-communicable diseases

The World Health Organization describes non-communicable diseases as diseases of long duration, generally slow progression and a major cause of adult mortality and morbidity. Non-communicable diseases (NCD), principally cardiovascular diseases, diabetes, cancers and chronic respiratory diseases, caused an estimated 35 million deaths in 2005, according to the WHO. This figure represents 60 per cent of all deaths globally, with 80 per cent of deaths due to non-communicable diseases occurring in low and middle income countries, and approximately 16 million deaths involving people under 70 years of age. A total of 63 per cent of all deaths in 2008 – 36 million people – were caused by NCDs. Total deaths from NCDs are projected to increase by a further 17 per cent over the next ten years.[1] The term non-communicable disease is a cause-based classification of disease. In this classification approach, diseases may be classified into three main groups: communicable disease, non-communicable disease and injuries. This is a predominantly research-based approach to disease classification, one based on causative agents. Non-communicable diseases are characterised by being non-infectious. However, being non-infectious does not mean being non-transmissible. The vectors for non-communicable diseases are not biological agents like mosquitoes, but social agents like alcohol, tobacco, unhealthy diet and physical inactivity. For example, comparison of diseases using this approach between Sub-Saharan Africa and the rest of the world is summarised in Figure 10.1.

Another approach to disease classification is an effect-based approach whereby all diseases are classified either as having acute or chronic effects. A majority of communicable diseases will be in the acute category, while most non-communicable disease will be classified as chronic. However, there are important exceptions. HIV and tuberculosis infections are essentially chronic infectious diseases, and they account for the bulk of chronic disease burden in Africa. Conversely, myocardial infarction and appendicitis are acute diseases despite not having an infectious aetiology. Some chronic diseases, such as emphysema, require regular acute care.

Infectious and chronic diseases interact with each other closely. For example, influenza is more likely to result in serious complications among individuals with pre-existing chronic diseases like chronic bronchitis or diabetes. Both infectious and chronic diseases are underpinned by common determinants of health such as poverty and poor housing. These two disease classification paradigms have led to inadequate attention being paid to the interface between infectious and chronic diseases in organisational capacity building efforts. Using an acute-chronic disease classification system, 76 per cent of all diseases in Sub-Saharan Africa in 2004 may be classified as chronic. A chronic disease classification is probably of greater utility to health planners, as conditions requiring long-term care place similar demands on patients, carers and health services, irrespective of their aetiology. Nevertheless, the non-communicable disease classification remains favoured by the academic community and the WHO.

Although not a major contributor to mortality, mental health conditions such as severe depression and schizophrenia contribute significantly to the global burden of diseases due to non-communicable disease. In 2002, 154 million people suffered from depression globally, 25 million people from schizophrenia and over 100 million people suffered from alcohol or drug abuse disorders. Close to 900,000 people die from suicide each year. Mental health conditions are also a substantial contributor to disability adjusted life years (DALY), contributing 13 per cent of all DALYs in 2004.[3] Mental health capacity building initiatives will be discussed in Chapter 14.

Diabetes, cardiovascular disease, chronic obstructive respiratory disease and cancers are the major categories of non-communicable diseases. Although not primarily caused by infections, their behavioural risk factors, such as tobacco, alcohol, physical activity and unhealthy diet are readily transferable from one population to another through global marketing and communication activities. The challenges of non-communicable disease to individuals, health systems and national economies are

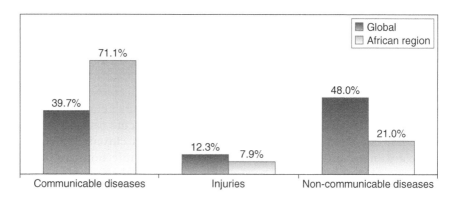

Figure 10.1 Distribution of burden of disease by per cent of total disability adjusted life years (DALY), 2004 (adapted from reference 2).

substantial. The World Bank estimates that deaths from NCDs as a share of total deaths are projected to rise by over 50 per cent in middle and lower income countries by 2030. The change will be particularly substantial in Sub-Saharan Africa, where NCDs will account for 46 per cent of all deaths by 2030, up from 28 per cent in 2008, and in South Asia, which will see the share of deaths from NCDs increase from 51 to 72 per cent during the same period (Figure 10.2).[3]

Cardiovascular diseases (CVD) and stroke constitute leading causes of morbidity and mortality from NCDs globally. Almost half of the 64 per cent of all deaths caused by NCDs globally in 2008 were attributable to CVD. Injuries accounted for 9 per cent of total global deaths, while communicable diseases, maternal and nutritional conditions accounted for the remaining 27 per cent of total deaths. About 10 per cent of the global burden of disease is attributable to CVD. At least 17 million people died from CVD in 2008. More than three million of these deaths occurred before the age of 60 and could have largely been prevented. The percentage of premature deaths from CVD ranges from 4 per cent in high income countries to 42 per cent in low income countries, leading to growing inequalities in the occurrence and outcome of CVDs between countries and populations.[5] In Australia, nearly 50,000 deaths were attributed to CVD in 2008. It was responsible for more deaths than any other disease group – 34 per cent of the total deaths for 2008. CVD accounted for about 18 per cent of the overall burden of disease in Australia in 2003, with coronary heart disease and stroke contributing over 80 per cent of this burden. CVD remains the most expensive disease group in Australia, costing about $5.9 billion in 2004–2005 with just over half of this money spent on patients admitted to hospital.[6]

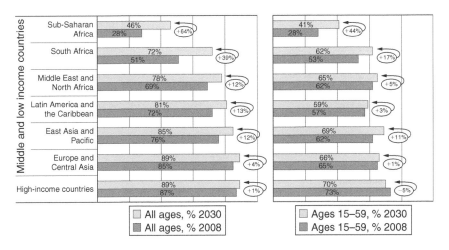

Figure 10.2 Deaths from NCDs as a share of total deaths (adapted from reference 4).

The major vectors of NCDs are tobacco, physical inactivity, alcohol and unhealthy diet. Tobacco use is associated with the deaths of six million people every year, or 10 per cent of total global deaths. Smoking causes an estimated 85 per cent of all lung cancer deaths in men and 80 per cent of all lung cancer deaths in women. An estimated 80 per cent of all deaths from chronic obstructive lung disease are related to tobacco smoking. Compared with non-smokers, smoking is estimated to increase the risk of coronary heart disease by two to four times, stroke by two to four times, men developing lung cancer by 23 times, women developing lung cancer by 13 times and dying from chronic obstructive lung diseases (i.e. chronic bronchitis and emphysema) by 12 times. Smoking is associated with cancers of blood cells (acute myeloid leukaemia), bladder, cervix, oesophagus, kidney, larynx, lung, tongue, pharynx, stomach and uterus. Smoking has many adverse reproductive and early childhood effects, including increased risk for infertility, pre-term delivery, stillbirth, low birth weight, osteoporosis and sudden infant death syndrome.[7]

Apart from health effects, NCDs have major adverse impacts on productivity. It is estimated that a 10 per cent increase in the prevalence of NCDs will precipitate a 0.5 per cent decline in gross domestic product. Addressing NCDs makes economic sense. A recent WHO report underlines that population-based measures for reducing tobacco and harmful alcohol use, as well as unhealthy diet and physical inactivity, are estimated to cost US$2 billion per year for all low and middle income countries, which in fact translates to less than US$0.40 per person.[8] The costs of NCDs on economies, individuals and health systems are shown in Figure 10.3.[9]

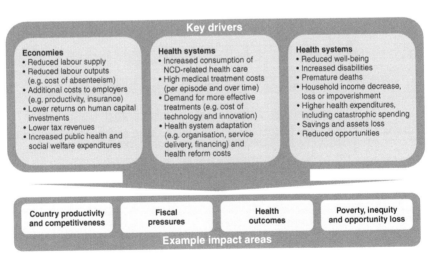

Figure 10.3 Effects of NCDs on economies, health systems and households (adapted from reference 9).

Capacity building for addressing social vectors of non-communicable disease

Tobacco

At an international level, the Tobacco Free Initiative (TFI) illustrates a global capacity building approach to address a prime risk factor for non-communicable disease. Established in July 1998, the mission of the TFI is to reduce the global burden of disease and death caused by tobacco, thereby protecting present and future generations from the devastating health, social, environmental and economic consequences of tobacco consumption and exposure to tobacco smoke. Its objectives are twofold; to ensure governments, international agencies and other entities are equipped effectively to implement national and transnational approaches to tobacco control in order to maximise the number of states becoming parties to and implementing the WHO Framework Convention on Tobacco Control (WHO FCTC) and, to increase the number of countries with effective tobacco control plans, policies and practices that take account of the provisions of the Convention. The capacity building approaches adopted by TFI stakeholders include; providing global policy leadership, encouraging mobilisation at all levels of society, promoting and supporting the WHO FCTC, encouraging countries to adhere to the WHO FCTC principles, supporting countries in efforts to implement tobacco control measures based on the WHO FCTC provisions, implementing surveillance and monitoring programmes, supporting and communicating empirical and behavioural research, and translating research. The FCTC is the world's first health treaty. It is already ratified by 171 nations as at mid-2011. It identifies policies that should help reduce tobacco use, such as stronger warning labels, smoke-free laws, advertising and promotion bans, and higher taxes.

Its evaluation indicates that significant demand exists, even in high smoking prevalence nations like China, for smoking cessation support, and that warning labels, higher taxes and probation of tobacco advertising are as effective in developed nations as they have been in selected poor nations, but that these policies are more difficult to implement in developing nations due, in part, to limited enforcement capacity. Evaluation also found that because warning labels on cigarettes constitute one of the limited sources of information about tobacco in low and middle income nations, they are more likely to be read by smokers in these countries compared with smokers in high income nations. However, although the potential is high, it is not optimised in nations like China and Malaysia, due to inconsistent enforcement and limited visibility of warning labels on cigarettes.[10]

An example of a global tobacco control capacity building initiative is that adopted by the Fogarty International Center (FIC) initiative's

International Tobacco and Health Research Capacity Building Program. This initiative builds tobacco control capacity based on three approaches: skill and tools development, building networks and leadership, and collection of local empirical data.[11]

Unhealthy diets

Unhealthy diets typically manifest clinically in underweight, overweight and micronutrient deficiencies. Each of these adverse manifestations has major consequences for NCDs. Low birth weight is associated with multiple factors, of which maternal undernutrition is a leading cause, particularly in developing nations. It appears that chronic diseases such as heart disease, stroke, diabetes, obesity, hypertension may be 'programmed' or gene functions modified, by inadequate or excessive supplies of energy or nutrients during pregnancy. Epigenetics, in relation to diet and non-communicable disease, is the inherited genome activity that does not depend on the naked DNA sequence. Epigenetics also explains how the same genotype can produce different phenotypes as it occurs in monozygotic twins.[12] Between 1980 and 2008, mean BMI worldwide increased by 0.4kg/m^2 per decade for men and 0.5kg/m^2 per decade for women. Male and female BMIs in 2008 were highest in some Oceania countries, reaching 33.9kg/m^2 (32.8–35.0) for men and 35.0kg/m^2 (33.6–36.3) for women in Nauru. Female BMI was lowest in Bangladesh (20.5kg/m^2, 19.8–21.3) and male BMI in Democratic Republic of the Congo 19.9kg/m^2 (18.2–21.5). Globally, mean BMI has increased since 1980. High BMI ($>30 \text{kg/m}^2$) denotes obesity, a factor associated with higher risk of NCDs such as heart disease and diabetes.[13]

Pacific Island countries such as Nauru and Tonga have among the highest rates of obesity globally, associated with high rates of diabetes and cardiovascular disease.[14]

Diets which are high in fat (especially saturated and trans fats), sugar and salt and low in fruits and vegetables increase the risk of developing NCDs. As the economies of Pacific nations change from subsistence agriculture to service and tourism industries, a change to such types of diets, often termed the nutrition transition, is being observed in most of these nations, and is an important factor in the rising rates of NCDs. For example, low fruit and vegetable intake is estimated to be a factor in 31 per cent of cardiovascular disease and 11 per cent of stroke cases worldwide. Countries, such as Japan and South Korea, which largely maintain traditional healthy cuisines despite increasing national wealth, have significantly lower burdens of non-communicable diseases.[15]

The scope for capacity building for addressing unhealthy diets is wide and complex (Figure 10.4).[16]

In July 2008, the city of New York became the first city in the United States to ban artery-clogging artificial trans fats at restaurants and public food outlets, and inform customers of the calorie content of foods served or

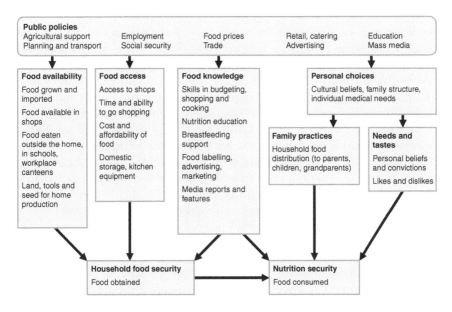

Figure 10.4 Capacity building entry points for addressing unhealthy diets.

sold. The United States Food and Drug Administration estimates the average American eats 4.7 lbs of trans fats each year. The trans fat prohibition initiative was strongly opposed by the restaurant industry as burdensome and unnecessary. The American Heart Association also opposed the New York Health Board initiative, claiming the ban may force eateries to revert to oils high in unhealthy saturated fats, such as butter. While current efforts at addressing unhealthy diets have focused on consumer education and medical treatment, New York's capacity building approach has focused on changing the make-up of food. The Department first undertook a voluntary campaign, but this effort did not decrease the proportion of restaurants that used artificial trans fats. By November 2008 – four months following the ban – estimated restaurant use of artificial trans fats for frying, baking or cooking or in spreads had decreased from 50 per cent to less than 2 per cent. Preliminary analyses suggest that replacement of artificial trans fats has resulted in products with more healthy fatty acid profiles. This initiative demonstrates that public health efforts that change food content to make default choices healthier enable consumers to more successfully reduce their cardiovascular risk. As at July 2011, Illinois became the fourteenth city to ban trans fats in food served in restaurants, movie theatres, cafes and bakeries or sold in school vending machines.[17] The October 2011 initiative by Denmark's government to introduce a tax on foods containing more than 3.25 per cent of saturated fats is complementary to the trans fats initiative, and will address the concerns of the American Heart Association.

Alcohol

An important starting point for alcohol use reduction is that no level of alcohol has been proven to be safe, and abstinence is key to avoiding alcohol-related harm.[18] Harmful alcohol consumption is estimated to be responsible for approximately 195,000 deaths a year in the European Union. Harmful alcohol use is the third biggest risk factor for early death and illness in the European Union, behind tobacco and high blood pressure.[19]

The Building Capacity project, with 31 country partners and ten European organisations, will support the EC in its public education on alcohol, helping to reduce the €125 billion of social costs due to alcohol each year in the European Union. It aims to build capacity at country, regional and municipal levels for effective programme and policy implementation through conferences and advocacy training events. In addition, the project seeks to undertake rigorous alcohol project reviews and document good practice to reduce binge drinking, drinking and driving, and improved consumer information through labelling and health warnings.[20] In Australia, alcohol is estimated to have contributed 3.2 per cent of the burden of disease in 2003. The inequality in the burden of alcohol-related disease is exemplified by the fact that alcohol contributed 6.2 per cent to the burden of disease among Indigenous Australians.

Capacity building for addressing alcohol-related morbidity and mortality needs to operate concurrently at primary, secondary and tertiary levels. Primary prevention interventions begin with prenatal and postnatal care, and include programmes that educate expectant parents on the risks of alcohol to the unborn child, such as Foetal Alcohol Spectrum Disorder. Secondary prevention interventions aim to prevent risky or problematic drinking, and avoid use developing into dependence. The main focus of tertiary prevention is treatment of alcohol and its health and social consequences. Capacity building efforts for addressing alcohol-related harm needs to co-opt communities affected by alcoholism in the design of alcohol harm minimisation programmes, and facilitate long-term partnerships with Indigenous community-controlled health organisations, and put in place strategies and time frames for handover of such alcohol control services to those organisations. Funding to address gaps in current capacity for tobacco control in vulnerable communities need to be identified and ameliorative processes funded accordingly.

Physical inactivity

Physical inactivity, defined as people undertaking 'insufficient' physical activity to achieve measurable health outcomes, is a strong risk factor for chronic diseases (Table 10.1).[21]

Physical inactivity can also contribute to other risk factors such as increases in blood pressure, blood cholesterol levels and overweight and obesity. There is strong evidence that a lack of regular physical activity is associated with an increased risk of mortality and morbidity from coronary heart disease. There is also some association between physical inactivity and an increase in risk of some types of stroke, heart failure and peripheral vascular disease. Insufficient physical activity increases the risk of Type 2 diabetes, osteoarthritis, osteoporosis, post-menopausal breast cancer and colorectal cancer. The Centers for Disease Control and Prevention (CDC) recommend that adults 'engage in moderate-intensity physical activity for at least 30 minutes on five or more days of the week', or 'engage in vigorous-intensity physical activity for at least 20 minutes on three or more days of the week'.[22] Determining the extent of physical activity is an important first step towards capacity building. In the United States, the CDC behavioural risk factor survey shows that although 76 per cent participate in some form of physical activity, only about 50 per cent of Americans engage in enough regular physical activity.[23] Capacity building approaches to improve physical activity rely on information, education and communication programmes. In Western Australia, for example, the Find Thirty Every Day® campaign aims to increase the number of West Australian adults who are sufficiently active for good health, by finding 30 minutes of physical activity every day.[24]

Given the significant cost of mass media campaigns for encouraging physical activity, evaluation research is important to evaluate the effectiveness of initiatives to improve physical activity. A systematic review to assess the effectiveness of interventions designed to improve physical activity

Table 10.1 Physical activity and chronic disease

Disease or condition	Risk factor					
	Tobacco smoking	Physical inactivity	Poor diet and nutrition	Excess body weight	High blood pressure	High blood cholesterol
Type 2 diabetes	–	✓	✓	✓	–	–
Asthma	✓	–	–	–	–	–
Coronary heart disease	✓	✓	✓	✓	✓	✓
Stroke	✓	✓	✓	✓	✓	✓
Lung cancer	✓	–	–	–	–	–
Colorectal cancer	–	✓	✓	✓	–	–
Osteoarthritis	–	✓	–	✓	–	–
Osteoporosis	✓	✓	–	–	–	–

Source: adapted from reference 21.

showed that two informational interventions ('point-of-decision' prompts to encourage stair use and community-wide campaigns) were effective, as were three behavioural and social interventions (school-based physical education, social support in community settings and individually adapted health behaviour change) and one environmental and policy intervention (creation of or enhanced access to places for physical activity combined with informational outreach activities) were effective.[25] Such studies guide capacity building efforts involving multi-disciplinary teams of health planners, architects and city developers.

Capacity building for cancer control

Cancer is a leading non-communicable disease cause of morbidity and mortality globally. In 2000, malignant tumours were responsible for 6.7 million (12 per cent) of the nearly 56 million deaths worldwide from all causes. In many countries, more than one-quarter of deaths are attributable to cancer. The WHO posits that if current trends continue, the estimated incidence of 12.7 million new cancer cases in 2008 will rise to 21.4 million by 2030, with nearly two-thirds of all cancer diagnoses occurring in low and middle income countries.[26] Capacity building for cancer control takes place at six main areas: research, prevention, early detection, treatment, patient welfare and cancer monitoring. Research into existing cancer prevention and treatment methods is an important consideration. Examples of positive research initiatives include the discovery and use of cervical cancer vaccine, *Helicobacter pylori* antibiotic treatment for prevention of stomach cancer, and hepatitis B vaccination for the prevention of liver cancer. Indeed, both environmental and social vectors account for over half of most new cancer cases, with the exception of breast cancer. Research studies which move towards intervention to reduce the impact of such vectors have been a major priority of global health agencies in the past two decades. For example, in relation to physical activity and cancer, research studies are required to generate accurate statistics on rates of inactivity and better statistics on which social groups are least active. Are people now less active because they don't have enough time to exercise? Or, is it because they spend so much time sitting in front of television sets and computers? Research is also needed on the types of activity that are best for different people, on what the best types of exercise programmes are, about the types of campaigns that will be most effective, and about how community amenities and local environments might be used to help people to be active in ways that are more convenient and enjoyable. Research studies into the genetic mechanisms of cancer are also required to improve early diagnosis and treatment options. Genetic research is providing new knowledge on the genetic changes which facilitate cancer progression of pre-malignant lesions of the oesophagus (Barrett's oesophagus).[27] Research studies into breast cancer associated genes

BRCA1 and BRCA2 have shown that both genes are inherited as auto-somal dominant mode and can be passed to offspring by either paternal or maternal lineage. In the general population the incidence of BRCA1 mutation is between 1 in 500 and 1 in 800. The most common mutation in BRCA1 is called 185delAG. It is located on chromosome 17, and the gene was cloned in 1994. This gene mutation is strongly associated with younger age of onset of breast cancer, and high grade malignancy. Such studies have built the evidence base and service delivery capacity for prophylactic bilateral mastectomy among high risk groups.[28]

Nearly 80 per cent of deaths attributable to NCDs occurred in low and middle income countries, where the highest proportions of deaths under the age of 70 years from these diseases occur. Preventing cancer needs to start from learning from successful initiatives implemented by developed nations to halt the incidence and prevalence of cancer. Occupational cancers are more common in developing countries, in part because most workplaces in developing countries are 'informal', i.e. they are not regularly surveyed or inspected, and laws for workers' protection are not implemented.[29] Strong regulatory controls, reliable data on occupational carcinogens and exposure prevention initiatives, worker education and constant attention to occupational health and safety issues are important capacity building measures in preventing occupational cancers. According to WHO guidelines, cancer prevention requires information on morbidity and mortality, identification of the most relevant causes and risk factors, where carcinogens are, how individuals become exposed, which are the most vulnerable groups, and what works better to eliminate or reduce the number of exposed or exposure levels.[29]

Addressing infectious risk factors for cancer, such as hepatitis B, hepatitis C, human papilloma virus and helicobacter pylori are important starting points. These infectious agents are responsible for up to 20 per cent of cancer incidence globally. Infectious agents also cause cancer in specific regions, such as in Egypt, *Shistosoma haematobium* and bladder cancer, and in parts of the Far East, Epstein-Barr virus and nasopharyngeal carcinoma. Building national and international capacities for vaccination, research into why and how these oncogenic agents evade the immune system and set up chronic infection, infection control programmes, screening and treatment are vital to address environmental vectors of cancer.[30]

The primary forms of cancer treatment are surgery, radiotherapy and chemotherapy. Each of these treatment modalities have been boosted by new technologies which enhance their specificity. For example, Dutch researchers recently discovered a tumour-specific fluorescent dye and an ultra-sensitive camera system that used during surgery can help surgeons identify difficult-to-spot ovarian cancers. The cancer cells literally glow, revealing themselves, so the surgeon can see what needs to be removed.[31]

The dye, which is linked to folate, could be used in up to 40 per cent of cancers, including kidney, lung, endometrial, colon and breast cancer.

Folate is a vitamin absorbed by cells, and ovarian cancer has one of the highest rates of folate receptor expression. This innovation is one of the research investments in nanomedicine. Biologically targeted radiotherapy in clinical practice requires a molecule which has a relative specificity for tumour tissue – the missile – coupled to a radionuclide with appropriate physical characteristics – the warhead. A precondition for the use of targeted radiotherapy is availability of customised computers to produce three-dimensional images of tumours being targeted. Current clinical studies in targeted radiotherapy focus on the integration of radionuclide treatment with conventional treatments, and the optimisation of such combined approaches. In 2011, preliminary findings from a phase 1 trial of a British study trialling targeted radio-immunotherapy for patients with Hodgkin's lymphoma showed inconclusive results. Radiation therapy has high recurrence rates for Hodgkin's lymphoma when used as the only form of treatment.[32] Targeted radiotherapy is expected to reduce the relatively high relapse rates.

Traditional chemotherapy drugs not only target cancer cells but kill healthy cells as well which is why they result in unpleasant side effects – such as sickness, fatigue, anaemia and hair loss. Molecularly targeted chemotherapy has addressed most of these side effects. Deregulation of kinase activity has emerged as a major mechanism by which cancer cells evade normal physiological constraints on growth and survival. Between 1995 and 2007 a family of molecularly targeted cancer chemotherapy called kinase inhibitors – used also in HIV chemotherapy – were almost three times more likely to be approved for use by patients than other types of anti-cancer drugs. As at June 2011, 11 kinase inhibitors have received US Food and Drug Administration approval as cancer treatments.[33]

Better understanding of a patient's genetic make-up and how they will respond to certain drugs has led to improvements in clinical trial design. Building appropriate capacity to improve cancer treatment using these three methods entail substantial investment in research and infrastructure. For example, to facilitate cancer research in regional and rural areas, infrastructural capacities which need to be developed include: physical infrastructure (such as, software, office space, office equipment or small pieces of research equipment to enable research), salary support (for example, funding of a full-time equivalent position for one year to enable time to be dedicated to research), staffing requirements (such as, part-time or full-time data managers, research assistants or pharmacists), training and education of staff (for example, attendance at a training course, relevant conferences or workshops), funding to enable linkages with a metropolitan health service for collaborative research purposes (such as, travel allowances or teleconference facilities) and funding to support regional workshops.

The recent Position Statement of 30 British cancer charities on the British government's proposed 2011 welfare reform bill illustrates a facet of patient welfare in relation to living with, or caring for someone with, cancer. The draft bill seeks to cut employment support allowance to individuals on cancer treatment after a maximum payment period of 12 months. The cancer charities' statement reads in part:

> The majority of people with cancer who are out of work want to return to work ... However, for many cancer patients it takes longer than a year to return to work. This is evident from your department's own statistics, which show that 75% of cancer patients who could be affected by this policy still need employment support allowance after one year.[34]

Other important aspects of cancer patients' welfare include participatory decision making and cultural competence of staff. Needs assessment of cancer patients' is an important prerequisite for capacity building in relation to holistic care. In *Approaching Death*, the Institute of Medicine identified key patient needs such as fears of abandonment and protracted death, and need for reliable, respectful care and advance care planning that promotes 'norms of decency'.[35]

Cancer monitoring occurs at patient and programme perspectives. At the cancer control programme level, cancer programme monitoring and evaluation entails determining whether a cancer control action plan is achieving its overall purpose of reducing the incidence and impact of cancer and reducing inequalities. It is also required to ensure that the various actions prescribed in the plan are meeting their expected outcomes, and that the milestones for each action are being achieved. Evaluation components at programme level include:

- *Formative evaluation*: evaluation in the early stages of implementation, where the evaluation itself contributes to implementation.
- *Process evaluation*: evaluation of systems and processes once a programme is up and running.
- *Output evaluation*: evaluating activities that result from the execution of a programme, but might not be termed outcomes at this stage.
- *Outcome evaluation*: sometimes referred to as summative evaluation, assesses whether the outcomes or results of a programme are consistent with the desired outcomes. An outcome evaluation study asks questions about whether the programme worked, and, if so, how well and for whom it worked.

In the United Kingdom, the 2011 National Health Service cancer strategy monitoring reveals that over 250,000 people in England are diagnosed with cancer every year and around 130,000 die from it. Currently, about 1.8 million people are living with and beyond a cancer diagnosis. Since April 2009, patients undergoing treatment for cancer, the effects of cancer or the effects of cancer treatment are entitled to exemption from prescription charges. Monitoring inequalities in cancer management is one of the core functions of the 2011 strategy. The report noted that:

> Incidence and mortality rates from cancer are higher in disadvantaged groups and areas, leading to worse outcomes and lowering our overall performance ... there is a range of inequalities in the outcomes and experience of cancer patients. These can occur at every stage of the patient pathway, including in awareness, incidence, access to treatment and care, patient experience, survival and mortality. They can also affect a range of groups in society, including socio-economically disadvantaged groups and areas, black and minority ethnic groups, older or younger people, men or women, people with disabilities, people from particular religions or with particular beliefs and the lesbian, gay, bisexual and transgender (LGBT) community.[36]

Capacity building activities for addressing inequalities in cancer care include the 2010 cancer patient experience survey, which revealed that younger people are the least positive about their experience, particularly around understanding completely what was wrong with them, and people with a disability or long-term condition reported a less positive experience than other patients across a wide range of issues measured in the survey. This was particularly marked for patients with a mental health condition or a learning disability.[36]

References

1 World Health Organization. *2008–2013 Action Plan for the Global Strategy for the Prevention and Control of Non-communicable Diseases.* Geneva: WHO, 2008.
2 World Health Organization. *Africa Health Statistics 2011.* Brazzaville: WHO Regional Office for Africa.
3 World Health Organization. *The Global Burden of Disease: 2004 Update.* Geneva: WHO, 2008.
4 World Bank. *The Growing Danger of Non-Communicable Diseases: Acting Now to Reverse Course.* Washington, DC: World Bank, 2011.
5 World Health Organization. *Global Atlas on Cardiovascular Disease Prevention and Control.* Geneva: WHO, 2011.
6 Australian Institute of Health and Welfare. *Cardiovascular Disease, Australian Facts, 2011.* Canberra: AIHW, 2011.
7 Centers for Disease Control. *Health Effects of Tobacco Smoking.* Atlanta, GA: CDC, 2010.
8 World Health Organization. *Global Status Report on Non-communicable Diseases 2010.* Geneva: WHO, 2011.
9 World Bank. Chronic emergency: why NCDs matter. Health, Nutrition, and Population Discussion Paper, Washington, DC: World Bank, 2011.
10 International Tobacco Control Policy Evaluation Project. The Framework Convention on Tobacco Control and the evaluation framework to support its

strong implementation: findings from the ITC Project. Waterloo, Ontario: ITC, 2009.

11 Stillman, F., Yang, G., Figueiredo, V., Hernandez, A.M., Samet, J. Building capacity for tobacco control research and policy. *Tobacco Control*, 2006; 15: i18–i23.

12 Esteller, M. Cancer epigenetics for the 21st century: what's next? *Genes and Cancer*, 2011; 2: 604–606.

13 Finucane, M.M., Stevens, G.A., Cowan, M.J. National, regional, and global trends in body-mass index since 1980: systematic analysis of health examination surveys and epidemiological studies with 960 country-years and 9.1 million participants. *Lancet*, 2011; 377: 557–567.

14 Ono, T., Guthold, R., Storng, K. *WHO Global Comparable Estimates*. Geneva: WHO, 2006.

15 World Health Organization. *Preventing Chronic Diseases: A Vital Investment*. Geneva: WHO, 2005.

16 World Health Organization. World Health Organization, World Health Assembly 55th meeting: global strategy on diet, physical activity and health. Resolution WHA55.23, 2002. Geneva: WHO, 2004.

17 Angell, S.Y., Silver, L.D., Goldstein, G.P., Johnson, C.M., Deithcher, D.R., Frieden, T.R., Bassett. M.T. Cholesterol control beyond the clinic: New York City's trans fat restriction. *Annals of Internal Medicine*, 2009; 151: 129–154.

18 Awofeso, N. Alcohol taxation policy in Australia: public health imperatives for action. *Medical Journal of Australia*, 2009; 190: 715–716.

19 European Commission. *Alcohol-related Harm in Europe: Key Data*. Brussels: EU, 2006.

20 European Union. *Building Capacity Project*. Ljubljana: Institute of Public Health of the Republic of Slovenia, 2011.

21 Australian Institute of Health and Ageing. *National Health Priority Area Risk Factors*. Canberra: AIHW, 2011.

22 National Center for Chronic Disease Prevention and Health Promotion and Centers for Disease Control and Prevention. *Preventing Obesity and Chronic Diseases through Good Nutrition and Physical Activity*. Atlanta, GA: CDC, 2008.

23 Centres for Disease Control. Behavioral risk factors surveillance survey. Available from: http://apps.nccd.cdc.gov/brfss/list.asp?cat=EX&yr=2010&qkey=4347 &state=All (accessed 23 November 2011).

24 Heart Foundation. *Find Thirty Every Day*. Perth: Heart Foundation, 2011.

25 Kahn, E.B., Ramsey, L.T., Brownson, R.C. The effectiveness of interventions to increase physical activity: a systematic review. *American Journal of Preventive Medicine*, 2002; 22: 73–107.

26 International Agency for Research on Cancer. Cancer incidence and mortality worldwide. Lyon: IARC Cancer Base No. 10, 2011.

27 Akagi, T., Ito, T., Kato, M., Jin, Z., Cheng, Y., Kan, T., *et al.* Chromosomal abnormalities and novel disease-related regions in progression from Barrett's esophagus to esophageal adenocarcinoma. *International Journal of Cancer*, 2009; 125: 2349–2359.

28 Rebbeck, T.R., Friebel, T., Lynch, H.T., Neuhausen, S.L., van't Veer, L., Garber. J.E., *et al.* Bilateral prophylactic mastectomy reduces breast cancer risk in *BRCA1* and *BRCA2* mutation carriers: the PROSE study group. *Journal of Clinical Oncology*, 2004; 22: 1055–1062.

29 Santana, V.S., Ribeiro, F.S.N. Occupational cancer burden in developing countries and the problem of informal workers. *Environmental Health*, 2011; 10 (Suppl. 1): S10.

30 Dalton-Griffin, L., Kellam, P. Infectious causes of cancer and their detection. *Journal of Biology*, 2009; 8: 67.

31 Dam, G.M.V., Themelis, G., Crane, L.M.A., Harlaar, N.J., Pleijhuis, R.G., Kelder, W., *et al.* Intraoperative tumor-specific fluorescence imaging in ovarian cancer by folate receptor-α targeting: first in-human results. *Nature Medicine*, 2011; 17: 1315–1319.
32 Meadows, A.T. Second cancers following Hodgkin's lymphoma: radiation therapy once more. *Annals of Oncology*, 2011; 22: 2569–2574.
33 Zhang, J., Yang, P.L., Gray, N.S. Targeting cancer with small molecule kinase inhibitors. *Nature Reviews Cancer*, 2009; 9: 28–39.
34 Cancer Charities UK. The welfare reform bill will affect people with cancer. *Guardian*, 9 March 2011. Available from: www.guardian.co.uk/politics/2011/mar/09/welfare-reform-bill-cancer (accessed 23 October 2011).
35 Field, M., Cassel, C. eds. Institute of Medicine. *Approaching Death: Improving Care at the End of Life*. Washington, DC: NAP, 1997.
36 National Health Service. *Improving Outcomes: A Strategy for Cancer*. London: NHS, 2011.

11 Capacity building for health systems research

Health systems research

Six interdependent health system building blocks are finance, workforce, services, technologies, information and governance. Four main functions of health systems are stewardship, financing, resource development and distribution, and service delivery. Research, in its broad sense, includes any gathering of data, information and facts for the advancement of knowledge. Health systems research may be described as the production of knowledge and applications to improve how societies organise themselves to achieve health goals. It includes how they plan, manage and finance activities to improve health, as well as the roles, perspectives and interests of different actors in this effort. Its main purpose is to produce scientific knowledge for the development of evidence-based policies and programmes towards equity, quality and efficiency in health.[1]

The 2004 Ministerial Summit on Health Research, held in Mexico, called for an enhancement of global health research with a focus on health systems, to achieve the health related Millennium Development Goals. An important objective of health systems research is to facilitate the use of evidence in policy making and health intervention. For example, whereas drugs to treat malaria are estimated to be 85 per cent effective, the community effectiveness of treatment among children is estimated to be only 3 per cent in Burkina Faso: only a small proportion of people with malaria attend health centres, and those who come receive low quality care, or do not all purchase and/or take the drugs as prescribed.[2] Health systems research focuses on developing practical approaches to address constraints to utilisation of health services and interventions. If such health systems barriers would be removed, related mortality would fall sharply. Health systems research has already made clear contributions to the knowledge about effective strategies to strengthen health systems. For example, while user fees were strongly advocated by various agencies during the 1980s as a means to overcome financial constraints, a 2008 publication reviewed current operational research studies and found that: (a) removing user fees increases the utilisation of curative, and in the longer term preventive, health care services; (b) although introduction of user fees may decrease health service utilisation, a combination of user fees and improvements in quality may increase utilisation. The authors decried the low quality of well-designed studies on the effect of user fees on service utilisation, in part due to inadequate funding of health systems research.[3] The two broad perspectives of types of research questions on user fees were summarised by Bennett *et al.* (Table 11.1).[4]

The research policy–implementation interface is complex, and strongly influenced by the stability and 'rationality' of social and institutional structures, congruity between 'official' and grassroots realities of health systems functioning, funding sources of research and programme implementation, relative under-valuation of research conducted using social science approaches as compared with biomedical approaches, and plurality of technical knowledge and perspectives. Health systems research has a broader domain and research utility compared with operational or implementation research.[5]

An important way of assessing regional activities in health systems research is by documenting scholarly publications in this field. International publications in health systems for industrialised countries doubled from 91,900 papers per year in 1991 to 178,800 in 2001. In less wealthy countries, however, human and financial resources have been insufficient to mount an effort that reflects the enormity of the knowledge gap. While yearly publications on developing countries have more than doubled, they have done so from a very low base of 3,900 in 1991 to 8,200 in 2001. South/north publication differentials thus point to a 5/95 gap in health systems research.[6] Of significance is the trend that the proportion of health systems research in developed nations have increased not only in absolute terms, but also in relation to the total research output, while the proportion of health systems research in relation to total research output has fallen sharply in developing nations (Figure 11.1).[7]

Capacity building approaches in research settings

Capacity building for health system research may be facilitated at four levels; funding of health services researchers and research, the focus of the research, the users of the research outputs and the utility of the research outputs. As most of the problems in relation to capacity building for health systems research are confined largely to developing nations, the bulk of discussions that follow relate to developing countries.

A lack of finance is undoubtedly a part of the reason why access to health services is not achieved for all in most developing countries. In most of Sub-Saharan Africa total health expenditure ranges from just US$4 per capita per year to about US$35 per capita per year, and much of this spending (~55 per cent) is private. The minimum cost of providing essential health services is estimated by the World Health Organization as US$40. While it is

Table 11.1 Possible policy implications of alternative types of research on user fees

Perspective	Typical research question	Illustrative policy implications
Positivist	What is the impact of user fees on service utilisation and across different groups of patients?	Levels at which user fees should be set. Which population groups should be exempt from fees?
Critical realist and relativist	Why were user fees introduced and how was equity conceived?	Strengthening the voice of the poor in policy and implementation processes so as to promote more pro-poor policies.
	How do out-of-pocket payments interact with other influences on care seeking?	Should policy focus on addressing user fees as the key obstacle to utilisation or would it also be necessary (or perhaps even more important) to address other barriers to care seeking?
	How is user fee policy experienced by those implementing it?	Strategies to empower health staff in the policy development and implementation processes, so as to ensure that the framing of policy takes account of their concerns, as a means to strengthening implementation.

Source: adapted from reference 4.

generally acknowledged that high quality health systems research is indispensable to improving efficiencies in health systems of developing nations, funding for health systems research has come in very small pots – with grants typically in the range of $20,000–30,000. With such limited funding it has been challenging to build research capacity in this area and almost impossible to undertake any major operational studies. High profile advocates are required to provide support for research to get its share of the national budgetary allocation in developing nations, and attract additional external funding. The current population of African researchers is ageing, and young talented researchers need to be identified early on in their careers. The inadequacy of career paths to attract and retain good researchers is the most serious impediment to health research. The development of attractive career pathways is key to bringing research in Sub-Saharan Africa to international standards of excellence. Capacity building in this regard may commence from clusters of centres of excellence, such as in the universities of Makerere (Uganda), Cape Town (South Africa) and Ibadan (Nigeria).[6]

The Commission on Macroeconomics and Health recommended the establishment of a Global Health Research Fund to provide US$1.5 billion per year for basic research on epidemiology, health economics and health systems research together with biomedical research. The commission recommends that health systems research expenditure should be about 2 per cent of total health expenditure.[8] International health research funding should be administered equitably, bearing in mind the unequal resource

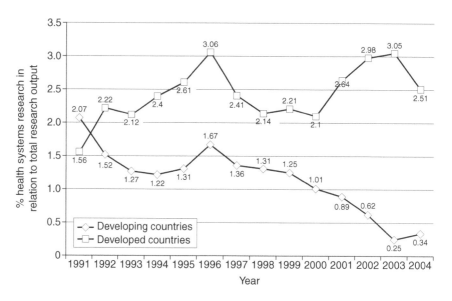

Figure 11.1 Health systems research output as percentage of total output in developing and developed nations, 1991–2004 (adapted from reference 7).

capabilities in health systems research between developing and developed nations. Funding for health systems research undertaken within developing countries was estimated by the Alliance for Health Policy and Systems Research at about US$134 million per annum in the period between 1999 and 2003. International donor funding accounted for about 69 per cent (US$92 million) of project funds, governments for 17 per cent (US$23 million) and the private sector for the remaining 14 per cent (US$18 million). As a whole, health systems research funds accounted for less than 0.5 per cent of total health expenditure – a big shortfall from the recommended 2 per cent level. Even as a percentage of all research, health systems research expenditure rates poorly. For example, in Colombia, of all the research projects undertaken between 1990 and 1997, 40 per cent were in the area of biomedical science, 29 per cent in clinical science, 23 per cent in epidemiology and only 8 per cent in health systems research. The Ministry of Health has not had a clear health systems research policy, or indeed a health research policy overall. As a result it has allocated research resources haphazardly. This is a vicious circle; if there is no policy to strengthen health systems research capacity it will be impossible to attain a critical mass of investigators and there will be no increase in the number of health systems research proposals for funding.[9]

Priority setting of health system research projects, including training, is a useful approach to substantially increase funding and to ensure efficient allocation, thus attracting more research funding to areas of greatest knowledge gaps. A 1998 survey by the WHO of more than 550 policy makers and almost 1,900 researchers in 13 low and middle income countries found that about one-third of policy makers, researchers and users of research interviewed said that there was either no rational process to set health research priorities in their country or that they were unaware of how priorities were identified or set.[10] Ideally, priority setting helps to focus health systems research and should be applied with the following considerations in mind: level at which research priorities should be set – i.e. local, national or international; comprehensiveness of research – e.g. exploratory or population-wide research studies; balance between technical (including quantitative) versus interpretive (including expert opinions and focus groups) approaches; and needs of stakeholders. Priority setting for disease prevention efforts is based, in part on burden of disease, community concern and international context.

For example, the burden of disease due to polio in Nigeria is much lower than that due to measles, but polio control was accorded higher priority from 2004 in line with global efforts to eradicate this disease by 2015. Priority setting in health systems research contexts involves value-laden choices, and technical approaches such as cost-effectiveness and burden of disease analyses do not equip decision makers to address a broader range of relevant values – such as trust, equity, accountability and fairness – that are of concern to other partners and, not least, the populations concerned. Developing adequate capacity to address these issues is important in identifying factors which result in inefficient use of health system resources. For example, patient satisfaction surveys of health services enable health managers to monitor this aspect of health service quality, and institute changes which are in keeping with sound customer orientation. In Western Australia, results of trends in patient satisfaction surveys from 2008 to 2011 are shown in Table 11.2.[11]

Capacity building for such health systems research entails the development of common validated survey instruments for use nationally, funding for periodic surveys, setting achievable action plans for 'root cause analysis' for adverse patient satisfaction survey trends, and using the data collected nationally and internationally to monitor this aspect of health care quality, which is not usually captured by conventional biomedical research methods. For example, in 2006, Health Policy Analysis Pty Ltd was engaged by the Steering Committee for the Review of Government Service Provision to review patient satisfaction and responsiveness surveys conducted in relation to public hospital services in Australia. The objectives of the review project were to identify points of commonality and difference between these patient satisfaction surveys and their potential for concordance and/or for forming the basis of a 'minimum national data set' on public hospital 'patient satisfaction' or 'patient experience', as well as identify data items in these surveys that could be used to report on an indicator of public hospital quality.[12] Such reviews are useful in establishing national and international best practice in relation to patient satisfaction in relation to hospital services in particular, and global patient responsiveness surveys in relation to health services in general.[13]

Table 11.2 Trends in patient satisfaction for patients admitted up to one month in Western Australia's hospitals

Scales, overall indicator of satisfaction and outcome score	2010–2011	2009–2010	2008–2009
Time and attention paid to patients' care	87.6	87.7	87.0
Meeting personal as well as clinical needs	91.0	91.2	90.6
Information and communication	84.0	84.0	83.3
Right to be involved in decisions about your care and treatment	71.4	70.5	70.8
Getting into hospital	68.1	67.3	64.0 ↓
Continuity of care	70.8	70.9	71.1
Residential aspects	62.7	63.4	62.9
Overall indicator of satisfaction	78.8	78.6	77.8 ↓
Outcome score	88.0	88.0	86.6 ↓

Source: adapted from Western Australia Health Department Annual Report, 2010–2011.

Notes
↓↑ Indicates that the mean scale score is statistically significantly lower or higher than the comparison score.

The potential users of health systems research are diverse, ranging from patient advocacy groups to policy makers, governments and international donor agencies. These users have differential access, particularly in developing nations, where access to computers and electronic databases is limited. To address such information asymmetry, many national and regional agencies are setting up customised health research databases, especially given that established systematic review databases explicitly favour randomised controlled trials over predominantly social sciences-based health systems research studies. In South Africa, for example, the National Health Research Database (NHRD), developed by the Health Systems Trust for the National Department of Health, is a web-based search engine and database that currently contains over 30,000 references, generally available as summaries/abstract, but, in addition, for many of the resources, there are links to full text PDF files of health research conducted in South and southern Africa.

The NHRD is also a tool for use at national and provincial level to receive and store health research protocols, unpublished literature and provide a low cost method of providing access to these. It is therefore an electronic repository for both formal and 'grey' literature. The primary purpose of the NHRD is to provide a central storage database for all health systems research conducted in South and southern Africa. Closely allied to this, is the NHRD's ability to function as a knowledge management tool for health systems research that is planned, produced, published or documented by both South African and other researchers conducting research in southern African communities and facilities. While the NHRD is accessible in the public domain, the primary users are intended to be research managers as well as researchers involved in conducting health research. These might range from researchers based at academic institutions to students conducting health research, government-based health managers, providers and policy makers.[14]

Another important capacity building approach to health systems research is improvement in Internet access in developing nations. With only 10 per cent of the population of developing nations having access to the Internet, and with access strongly influenced by urban residence and wealth status, the current digital divide is more intense than inequities in health or income. Given the paucity of health systems research in Africa, access to quality published studies in other developing nations as well as in developed nations is important. A major constraint on access to research publications is the high commercial online subscription costs for many journals. The WHO enables free access to full text articles in low income countries via the Health Internetwork Access Research Initiative programme (HINARI).[15] Over 80 publishers, including Blackwell Science and John Wiley contribute content to HINARI. Capacity building components of the HINARI initiative include trainers' workshops, and technical support. Alternative models for building capacity to access health systems research include reduced journal costs negotiated with publishers, and open access journals.

The utility of health systems research output is critically dependent on the extent to which such research is translated to policy and practice. However, unlike clinical research findings, whose translation is well supported by pharmaceutical companies and government agencies, health systems research receives comparatively little support. Unlike new drug discoveries, there is less compelling pressure from patients, industry or health workers for health managers to implement translational research findings. Capacity building for improving utility of health systems research need to address three drivers. First, improving the understanding of the dynamics of diffusion of innovation, as well as social science techniques for translating research findings, such as 'positive deviance' and 'social marketing' techniques.[16] Second, encourage inter-professional training, so that researchers and policy makers are 'on the same page' with regards to the linkages and networks for enhancing the utility of research output. In most nations currently, basic scientists are not generally trained to think of the clinical application of their work, clinicians are often not taught to formulate research studies based on clinical observations and public health scientists may not have a strong background in basic or clinical research (but have the knowledge of the community the other two groups may lack). Capacity building to break down the silos between these three groups and encourage the development of a seamless process to replace the T1, T2 and T3 paradigms is a useful approach to improve research utility. Third, provide evidence of the need and overall effectiveness for change, even if such change is not as targeted as with clinical research translation.

A major encumbrance to translating health systems research into policy is the 'prevention paradox', whereby the high risk groups do not necessarily have the highest burden of disease or constitute the highest threat to public health. Many health systems interventions that aim to improve health have relatively small influences and perceptible benefits on the health of most people. Therefore for one person to benefit, many people have to change their behaviour – even though they receive no benefit, or even may even suffer, from the change.[17] Thus, policy makers have a greater obligation to demonstrate value for money for health systems evidence-based policies. Fortunately, there are a variety of tools to demonstrate the need for such research-based policy implementation, such as information, education and communication programmes, in addition to the more clinically oriented randomised controlled trials and cost-effectiveness analyses.

References

1 Varkevisser, C., Brownlee, A., Pathmanathan, I. *Handbook on Health Systems Research*, 2nd ed. Amsterdam, KIT/IDRC, 2003.
2 Krause, G., Sauerborn, R. Comprehensive community effectiveness of health care: a study of malaria treatment in children and adults in rural Burkina Faso. *Annals of Tropical Paediatrics*, 2000; 20: 273–282.

3 Lagarde, M., Palmer, N. The impact of user fees on health service utilization in low- and middle-income countries: how strong is the evidence? *Bulletin of the World Health Organization*, 2008; 86: 839–848.

4 Bennett, S., Agyepong, I.A., Sheikh, K., Hanson, K., Ssengooba, F., Gilson, L. Building the field of health policy and systems research: an agenda for action. *PLoS Medicine*, 2011; 8: e1001081.

5 Remme, J.H.F., Adam, T., Becerra-Posada, F., D'Arcangues, C., Devlin, M., Gardner, C., *et al.* Defining research to improve health systems. *PLoS Medicine*, 2010; 7: e1001000.

6 Whitworth, J.A.G., Kokwaro, G., Kinyanjui, S., Snewin, V.A., Tanner, M., Walport, M., Sewankambo, N. Strengthening capacity for health research in Africa. *Lancet*, 2008; 372: 1590–1593.

7 Gonzalez, B.M., Mills, A. Assessing capacity for health policy and systems research in low and middle income countries. *Health Research Policy and Systems*, 2003; 1: 1–20.

8 Macroeconomics and Health. Investing in health for economic development. Report of the Commission for Macroeconomics and Health. Geneva: WHO, 2001.

9 Alliance for Health Policy and Systems Research. *Strengthening Health Systems: The Role and Promise of Policy and Systems Research.* Geneva: WHO, 2004.

10 Working Group on Priority Setting. Priority setting for health research: lessons from developing countries. *Health Policy and Planning*, 2000; 15: 130–136.

11 Department of Health, Western Australia. *Patient Evaluation of Health Services.* Perth: Western Australia, 2011.

12 Pearse, J. Review of patient satisfaction and experience surveys conducted for public hospitals in Australia. A Research Paper for the Steering Committee for the Review of Government Service Provision. Sydney: Health Policy Analysis Pty, 2005.

13 World Health Organization. *World Health Survey 2002: Patient Responsiveness Survey.* Geneva: WHO, 2002.

14 Department of Health, Republic of South Africa. South African National Health Research Database, Pretoria, South Africa, 2011.

15 World Health Organization. *Health Internetwork Research Access Initiative.* Geneva: WHO, 2009.

16 Awofeso, N. Implementing smoking cessation programs in prison settings. *Addiction Research and Theory*, 2003; 11: 118–130.

17 Caetano, R., Mills, B.A. The Hispanic Americans baseline alcohol survey (HABLAS): is the 'prevention paradox' applicable to alcohol problems across Hispanic national groups? *Alcohol Clinical and Experimental Research*, 2011; 35: 1256–1264.

12 Capacity building for health workforce and services delivery

Health workforce trends

The 2006 *World Health Report* defines health workers as all paid workers in health organisations or institutions whose primary intent is to improve health as well as those whose personal actions are primarily intended to improve health but who work for other types of organisations. Based on this definition, it is estimated that there were 59.2 million full-time paid health workers worldwide in 2005 (Table 12.1).[1]

WHO has identified a threshold in workforce density below which high coverage of essential interventions, including those necessary to meet the health-related Millennium Development Goals (MDGs), is very unlikely. This threshold is based on 0.5 doctors, 1.5 nurses and 0.8 midwives per 1,000 population. Countries with a combined basic workforce quantity of less than 2.28 doctors, nurses and midwives per 1,000 population are classified as having a severe shortage of health workers. Based on this modelling, it was determined that, as at 2006, there were 57 countries with critical health workforce shortages, equivalent to a global deficit of 2.4 million doctors, nurses and midwives. The proportional shortfalls are greatest in Sub-Saharan Africa, although numerical deficits are very large in Southeast Asia because of its population size.

The health workforce extends far beyond the WHO's modelling formula, and includes dentists, public health workers, pharmacists, physiotherapists, health managers and laboratory technicians. Training of health workforce is the primary mechanism for building capacity to optimise the quantity of health workers. Assuring adequate quantity of health workers is thus highly dependent on the quality of basic and tertiary education in a given country, attractiveness of health professions in relation to other disciplines, management of losses through attrition, migration, retirement and death, and health worker additions through NGO-affiliated health workers, and employment of overseas health professionals. A recent modelling study asserted that numerical inadequacy of health workers has become 'the binding constraint in implementing many priority health programs in Africa'.[2]

Table 12.1 Global health workforce by density

WHO region	Total health workforce		Health services providers		Health management and support workers	
	Number	Density (per 1,000 population)	Number	Percentage of total health workforce	Number	Percentage of total health workforce
Africa	1,640,000	2.3	1,360,000	83	280,000	17
Eastern Mediterranean	2,100,000	4.0	1,580,000	75	520,000	25
South-East Asia	7,040,000	4.3	4,730,000	67	2,300,000	33
Western Pacific	10,070,000	5.8	7,810,000	78	2,260,000	23
Europe	16,630,000	18.9	11,540,000	69	5,090,000	31
Americas	21,740,000	24.8	12,460,000	57	9,280,000	43
World	59,220,000	9.3	39,470,000	67	19,750,000	33

Source: adapted from reference 1.

The quality of primary and secondary education is just above average in Africa. An emerging trend in this regard is the inferior completion rate of males relative to females in most nations, as well as ethnic differences. In the United States, a 2006 report titled; *Leaving Boys Behind: Public High School Graduation Rates*,[3] found that, in 2003, 59 per cent of African-American girls, but only 48 per cent of African-American boys, earned their diplomas that year. Among Hispanics, the graduation rate was 58 per cent for girls, but only 49 per cent for boys. Similar trends have been observed in Africa and Asia. This trend has important implications for capacity building for future health professionals. The MDG targets on education and gender parity are based on the assumption that boys are preferenced in relation to education. Hence it is very likely that these MDG targets will be met without adequately addressing the important issue of low educational enrolment and quality. For example, India's government proudly announced in its 2009 MDG report that it achieved gender parity in primary and secondary education in 2004. What this target attainment appears to ignore is that 27 per cent of India's population are not completing high school, since female enrolment only matched the 73 per cent male high school completion rate documented for 2004.[4] Thus, more sensitive indicators of the quality of secondary school education are required in building capacity for future skilled health workforce in developing nations.

Training of health workers is expensive, and the countries with the most severe shortage have the least adequate training infrastructure. To take the example of graduate public health training, only 8 per cent of Portuguese-speaking African countries, and 66 per cent of Francophone African nations have tertiary public health training capacity. For a population of 900 million people, there are fewer than 600 full-time academic public health staff in tertiary institutions.[5]

Capacity building for optimising health workforce

The critical shortage in Africa's public health education capacity applies to other health disciplines, and to other developing nations. There are several options to improve capacity for increasing the quantity of health workers. First, development cooperation agreements may be utilised to allow wealthy nations to fund the establishment and staffing of health training schools. This is the approach adopted by Zambia. The THET (Tropical Health and Education Trust) was established in 1988 by Professor Eldryd Parry, to address the substantial needs of medical schools and hospitals in developing countries. In particular, it became necessary to respond to the significant gaps in undergraduate and postgraduate health education – nursing, midwifery, pharmacy, laboratory science and many other disciplines. THET has been appointed the management agent for a project aimed at strengthening the capacity of Zambia health training institutions to train health workers. This is funded by the UK Department for International Development (DFID), but has had significant support from the Department of Health, which provided support for the initial scoping of the proposal. The outcome of the capacity building initiative was a revitalisation of the University of Zambia medical school, with the DFID providing international academics as part of an Overseas Development Assistance funding. Salaries of Zambian health training staff and frontline health workers were tripled, and the increases were funded by international aid from the United Kingdom's foreign aid programme. The School of Medicine, University of Zambia, has been successful in establishing Master of Medicine programmes in a number of postgraduate medical specialities including surgery, orthopaedics, urology, obstetrics and gynaecology, paediatrics and general medicine. Retention of fully trained doctors in Zambia has improved significantly with this strategy.[6]

A related strategy is overseas recruitment of health workers. In countries like Maldives which have no medical school, overseas recruitment is a major strategy for improving the quantity of health workers. Overseas recruitment of health workers may also provide a temporary strategy for countries such as Australia, the United States and Saudi Arabia, which are accelerating efforts to train local health workers to address current health workforce shortages. These recruitments have provided critical workforce to rural areas of these countries, where local health workers are generally unwilling to work in. For example, the US Department of Health and Human Services (HHS) estimated that the United States weathered a shortfall of 275,000 full-time equivalent registered nurses in 2010. During the past 50 years the United States has regularly imported nurses to ease its nurse shortages. Although the proportion of foreign nurses had never exceeded 5 per cent of the US nurse workforce until 1990, that proportion rose to 14 per cent in 2004.[7] It is noteworthy that this strategy is expensive, and thus only affordable by low and middle income countries. In poor countries like Haiti and South Sudan, NGOs have helped address health workers' shortage by setting up long-term aid projects financed by donors. For example, Médecins Sans Frontières' (MSF) hospital programme in Agok, South Sudan, provides a wide range of care including surgical, maternity, inpatient and outpatient care, and includes a paediatric unit, a tuberculosis ward and a therapeutic feeding centre for malnourished children. This hospital is staffed mainly by health workers employed and paid by MSF.

A third, but so far underutilised, approach for increasing the quantity of health workers is through distance education for tertiary education. Given the high cost of establishing and staffing tertiary health training institutions, open and distance learning programmes provide efficient opportunities to build adequate workforce capacity. The terms *open learning* and *distance education* represent approaches that focus on opening access to education and training provision, freeing learners from the constraints of time and place, and offering flexible learning opportunities to individuals and groups of learners. The potential impact of open and distance learning on all education delivery systems has been greatly accentuated through the development of Internet-based information technologies. Capital investments usually substitute for high recurrent costs, making economies of scale a decisive factor for efficiency savings with open and distance learning.

An example of open and distance learning in tertiary health training is the Peoples-uni open access education initiative. The goal of Peoples-uni is 'to contribute to improvements in the health of populations in low- to middle-income countries by building Public Health capacity via e-learning'. Its objectives are: (1) to provide public health education for those working in low to middle income countries who would otherwise not be able to access such education, via Internet based e-learning; (2) to utilise a 'social model' of capacity building, with volunteer academic and support staff and 'open educational resources' available through the Internet, using a collaborative approach and modern information and communication technology (ICT); (3) to offer education at the 'train the trainers' level, equivalent to that of a Master's degree, for those with prior educational and occupational experience; (4) the education will meet identified competences which help with the evidence-based practice of public health and be action oriented, to assist in tackling major health problems facing the populations in which the students work; (5) create an educational portfolio leading to a Certificate and Diploma in Public Health based on being shown to have met the competences identified in course modules, and an upgrade to the Master of Public Health based on further work. Established in 2007, Peoples-uni runs three semesters, with more than 100 students each time. Students have come from 30 countries, and volunteer tutors and support group from 22 countries. Situation analyses already performed suggest that the need for this education is great and that this solution may be feasible in many countries.[8]

Globally, approximately one-half of the population lives in rural areas, but less than 38 per cent of the nurses and less than 25 per cent of the physicians work there. While getting and keeping health workers in rural and remote areas is a challenge for all countries, nations already experience absolute shortage of health workers. In 2010, the World Health Organization released a strategy document for assuring retention and equitable distribution of health workers. These strategies were categorised as education (e.g. design of continuing education and professional development programmes that meet the needs of rural health workers and that are accessible from where they live and work, so as to support their retention), regulatory (e.g. introduce and regulate enhanced scopes of practice in rural and remote areas to increase the potential for job satisfaction, thereby assisting recruitment and retention), financial incentives (e.g. use a combination of fiscally sustainable financial incentives, such as hardship allowances, grants for housing, free transportation, paid vacations, sufficient enough to outweigh the opportunity costs associated with working in rural areas, as perceived by health workers, to improve rural retention), personal and professional support (improve living conditions for health workers and their families and invest in infrastructure and services such as sanitation, electricity, telecommunications and schools, as these factors have a significant influence on a health worker's decision to locate to and remain in rural areas).[9]

Distribution variances of health workforce are normally viewed essentially as rural–urban divides, with health workers more likely to work in urban areas. Such imbalance is most pronounced in developed nations, where rural infrastructure and social services are too basic to support the lifestyles of tertiary educated workforce and their families. The resulting imbalance has major implications for the quality of health services and health outcomes. In Indonesia, for example, 0.9 million eligible children missed measles vaccination, and 19,456 cases of measles were documented among Indonesian children in 2007. Analysis of Indonesia's Demographic and Health Survey 2007 data revealed that the first-dose measles vaccination coverage in rural areas of Indonesia was 68.5 per cent, compared with 80.1 per cent in urban regions ($p < 0.001$).[10] A significant health worker shortage situation exists in Indonesia, and the shortage is more pronounced in rural areas.[11] Similar rural health worker shortfalls have been reported in industrialised nations.[12] In Australia, workforce capacity building strategy is aimed at 'improved capacity, quality and mix of the health workforce to meet the requirements of health services, including through training, registration, accreditation and distribution strategies'. The average number of full-time equivalent Australian-based GPs per 100,000 population varies from a peak of over 100 in the best serviced cities, to as low as 25.3 in very remote areas. The average number of medical workers varies from over 600 in the best serviced cities to a low of 30 in very remote areas. One of the capacity building initiatives in relation to improving distribution of health workers is provision of incentives for health professionals' education, complemented with bonded rural scholarships for core health workers, who would be required to work in underserved areas following graduation. Following this initiative, the numbers of core health professionals have increased substantially.[13]

In conjunction with short- to medium-term employment of overseas-trained doctors and nurses, these strategies have been largely successful in addressing health worker distribution. Other approaches to capacity building to improve health workforce capacity include the creation of specialised cadres such as assistant doctors and nurse practitioners, as well as task-shifting, which enables other health workers to undertake tasks traditionally reserved for doctors and nurses. When adequate capacity building processes are undertaken during the implantation phase, outcomes of care are generally comparable to those delivered by cadres traditionally entrusted with such responsibilities. For example, a US study comparing clinical outcomes delivered by nurse practitioners and physicians found:

> In an ambulatory care situation in which patients were randomly assigned to either nurse practitioners or physicians, and where nurse practitioners had the same authority, responsibilities, productivity and administrative requirements, and patient population as primary care physicians, patients' outcomes were comparable.[14]

References

1 World Health Organization. *The World Health Report 2006: Working Together for Health.* Geneva: WHO, 2006.

2 Scheffler, R.M., Mahoney, C.B., Fulton, B., Dal Poz, M.R., Preker, A.S. Estimates of health care professional shortages in sub-Saharan Africa by 2015. *Health Affairs,* 2009; 28: w849–w862.

3 Greene, J.P., Winters, W.A. *Leaving Boys Behind: Public High School Graduation Rates.* New York: Manhattan Institute for Policy Research, 2006.

4 UNESCO. *Educational Statistics, India, 2004.* Paris: UNESCO, 2008.

5 IJsselmuiden, C.B., Nchinda, T.C., Duale, S., Tumwesigye, N.M., Serwadda, D. Mapping Africa's advanced public health education capacity: the AfriHealth project. *Bulletin of the World Health Organization,* 2007; 85: DOI 10.2471/ BLT.07.045526.

6 Department for International Development. *Evaluation of Country Programs: Zambia.* London: DFID, 2008.

7 Brush, B.L., Sochalski, J., Berger, A.M. Imported care: recruiting foreign nurses to U.S. health care facilities. *Health Affairs,* 2004; 23: 78–87.

8 Heller, R.F., Chongsuvivatwong, V., Hailegeorgios, S., Dada, J., Torun, P., Madhok, R., Sandars, J. People's Open Access Education Initiative. Capacity-building for public health: http://peoples-uni.org. *Bulletin of the World Health Organisation,* 2007; 85: 901–980.

9 World Health Organization. *Increasing Access to Health Workers in Remote and Rural Areas through Improved Retention: Global Policy Recommendations.* Geneva: WHO, 2010.

10 Fernandez, R.C., Awofeso, N., Rammohan, A. Determinants of apparent rural–urban differentials in measles vaccination uptake in Indonesia. *Rural and Remote Health,* 2011; 11: 1702 (online).

11 Rokx, C., Giles, J., Satriawan, E., Marzoeki, P., Harimurti, P., Yavuz, E. New *Insights into the Provision of Health Services in Indonesia: A Health Workforce Study.* Washington, DC: International Bank for Reconstruction and Development/ World Bank, 2010.

12 MacDowell, M., Glasser, M., Fitts, M., Nielsen, K., Hunsaker, M. A national view of rural health workforce issues in the USA. *Rural and Remote Health,* 2010; 10: 1531 (Online).

13 Commonwealth of Australia. *Health Workforce Strategy 12.* Canberra: ADHA, 2010.

14 Mundinger, M.O., Kane, R.L., Lenz, E.R., Totten, A.M., Tsai, W.-Y., Cleary, P.D., *et al.* Primary care outcomes in patients treated by nurse practitioners or physicians: a randomized trial. *Journal of American Medical Association,* 2000; 283: 59–68.

13 Capacity building for reducing maternal mortality

Maternal mortality reduction: two centuries of progress

The major definitions and measures of maternal mortality are: *maternal death* – the death of a woman while pregnant or within 42 days of termination of pregnancy, irrespective of the duration and site of the pregnancy, from any cause related to or aggravated by the pregnancy or its management, but not from accidental or incidental causes (ICD-10); *maternal mortality ratio* – number of maternal deaths during given time period per 100,000 live births during same time period; *maternal mortality rate* – number of maternal deaths in given time period per 100,000 women of reproductive age, or woman-years of risk exposure, in same time period; *lifetime risk of maternal death* – probability of maternal death during a woman's reproductive life, usually expressed in terms of odds; *proportionate mortality ratio* – maternal deaths as proportion of all female deaths of those of reproductive age, usually defined as 15–49 years in a given time.[1]

Maternal mortality is a major cause of maternal and infant deaths. Two centuries ago, 2 per cent of all pregnancies resulted in a maternal death, similar to what obtains in some regions of northern Nigeria and Afghanistan currently. Most of these deaths occurred around the time of delivery, and resultant pregnancy loss was common. Data on historical trends in maternal mortality in countries with the highest burden are scarce. In England and Wales, formal record keeping of deaths in childbirth commenced in 1847. The maternal mortality ratio in 1856–1860, for example, was 460/100,000. Prior midwifery records dating back to 1780 showed a range in maternal mortality ratio of between 100/100,000 and 600/100,000. From the 1930s, maternal mortality ratio in the United Kingdom showed a steep decline,[2] and was 8.2/100,000 live births in 2010. This trend was attributed to higher living standards, infection control, and improved medical care, especially from the 1940s onwards globally, the number of maternal deaths dropped from more than 500,000 a year in 1980 to 343,000 a year in 2008. The lifetime risk of maternal deaths vary from one in 4,300 in industrialised nations to one in 37 in the least developed nations. The global lifetime risk of maternal death is one in 140.

Infections, and particularly puerperal sepsis, were a common cause of maternal mortality in the pre-antibiotic era. Immediately postnatally, the placental site is a large open wound – easily invaded by ascending bacteria. Sepsis following delivery was responsible for up to 40 per cent of maternal death. For centuries, it was recognised that puerperal women were at risk of a fever that could be fatal. Dr Ignaz Semmelweis was the first to identify the mode of transmission of puerperal sepsis. He conducted studies on maternity data available at Allgemeines Krankenhaus in Austria and Dublin Maternity Hospital in Ireland (1784–1858). He found that male obstetricians and medical students who conducted autopsies inadvertently transferred infection to women during delivery. Introduction of chlorine handwashing reduced puerperal sepsis. Although he was confident about the potential of his findings to reduce maternal mortality globally, as may be inferred from his 1861 statement; 'My doctrine is produced in order to banish the terror from lying-in hospitals, to preserve the wife to the husband, and the mother to the child', he was shunned by the medical establishment and died from torture wounds while being detailed in a psychiatric hospital in 1865.[3] From around 1880, Listerian antisepsis was gradually introduced into obstetrics, which significantly reduced maternal mortality.[4]

The declines in maternal mortality were not uniform globally. While maternal deaths became a rarity in developed nations – in Australia, deaths from puerperal sepsis are extraordinarily rare (the MMR is currently about 0.1 per 1,000 births) – it is still a major cause of female and infant deaths in the developing world. The 2000 Millennium Development Goal 5 has two targets focussed on reducing maternal mortality: 'Target 5.A. Reduce by three quarters, between 1990 and 2015, the maternal mortality ratio', 'Target 5.B. Achieve, by 2015, universal access to reproductive health.'[5] Preliminary data from a 2010 World Health Organization review of global causes of maternal mortality are shown in Table 13.1.

Of all the MDGs, the least progress has been made on the maternal health goal – worldwide, the maternal mortality ratio declined at a rate of less than 1 per cent from 1990 to 2005.

According to World Bank statistics, although there was a 35 per cent decrease in maternal deaths from 1990 to 2008, only 13 per cent of nations (23 out of 181) are on track to reduce maternal mortality by 75 per cent compared with 1990 levels. Ten out of 87 countries with maternal mortality ratios equal to or over 100 in 1990 are on track with an annual decline of 5.5 per cent between 1990 and 2008. At the other extreme, 30 countries made insufficient or no progress in maternal mortality reduction since 1990.[6,7]

In a 2010 report, the WHO stated that the number of women dying due to complications during pregnancy and childbirth has decreased by 34 per cent from an estimated 546,000 in 1990 to 358,000 in 2008. However, the remarkable progress is insufficient to achieve the MDG of reducing

Table 13.1 WHO preliminary data on the causes of maternal mortality globally

Indicator	Acceptable level
1 Availability of emergency obstetric care: basic and comprehensive care facilities	There are at least 5 emergency obstetric care facilities (including at least 1 comprehensive facility) for every 500,000 population
2 Geographical distribution of emergency obstetric care facilities	All subnational areas have at least 5 emergency obstetric care facilities (including at least 1 comprehensive facility) for every 500,000 population
3 Proportion of all births in emergency obstetric care facilities	(Minimum acceptable level to be set locally)
4 Met need for emergency obstetric care: proportion of women with major obstetric complications who are treated in such facilities	100% of women estimated to have major direct obstetric complication are treated in emergency obstetric care facilities
5 Caesarean sections as a proportion of all births	The estimated proportion of births by caesarean section in the population is not less than 5% or more than 15%
6 Direct obstetric case fatality rate	The case fatality rate among women with direct obstetric complications in emergency obstetric care facilities is less than 1%

Source: UNICEF (public domain), available from http://www.childinfo.org/facts_1231.htm (accessed 2 April 2011).

maternal mortality by 75 per cent by 2015. This will require an annual decline of 5.5 per cent. The 34 per cent decline since 1990 translates into an average annual decline of just 2.3 per cent. The report highlighted that pregnant women still die from four major causes: severe bleeding after childbirth, infections, hypertensive disorders and unsafe abortion. Every day, about 1,000 women died due to these complications in 2008. Out of the 1,000, 570 lived in Sub-Saharan Africa, 300 in South Asia and five in high income countries. The risk of a woman in a developing country dying from a pregnancy-related cause during her lifetime is about 36 times higher compared to a woman living in a developed country.[8] Investing in better maternal health not only improves a mother's health and that of her family, but also increases the number of women in the workforce and promotes the economic well-being of communities and countries. Untreated pregnancy and birth complications mean that at least ten million women become disabled every year, undermining their ability to support their families.[7]

Strategies for reducing maternal mortality

An eight-pronged strategy is suggested for improving maternal health and reducing maternal mortality:

- *enhance* the quality, quantity and distribution of emergency obstetric facilities and workforce, in order to reduce perinatal maternal and child deaths;
- *develop* more effective and efficient national health systems;
- *motivate* young people to delay pregnancy and achieve higher levels of education;
- *support* increased use of reproductive health services, focussing on assisted deliveries and family planning;
- *tie* financing to performance in maternal health programmes;
- *protect* poor women from ill health and unaffordable costs and treatment;
- *identify* and promote best practice programmes to reduce maternal ill health and death;
- *build* adequate capacity in workforce and infrastructure to address maternal mortality's causes, particularly among vulnerable populations.

All pregnant women are at risk of obstetric complications. Most life-threatening complications occur during labour and delivery, and these cannot all be predicted. Prenatal screening does not identify all of the women who will develop complications. Women not identified as 'high risk' can and do develop obstetric complications. Most obstetric complications occur among women with no risk factors. Thus, *emergency obstetric care* is an essential component in reducing maternal mortality and improving pregnancy outcomes. Emergency obstetric care includes specific interventions to manage emergency obstetric complications. Interventions may be intravenous antibiotics, oxytocics or anti-convulsants, management of abortion complications, management of postpartum bleeding, assisted delivery for prolonged labour such as vacuum or forceps delivery, blood transfusion and/or caesarean section.[9] A 2009 report on emergency obstetric care up scaling published by the WHO lists the indicators of basic compliance (see Table 13.2).

Programmes for maternal and child health improvements, and maternal mortality reductions, are best undertaken within the framework of a well-functioning health system. Countries like Sri Lanka and Malaysia which have invested in health system strengthening have reaped huge rewards in relation to improvements in maternal and child health.[11] The health systems of the worst performing nations in terms of maternal mortality reduction, such as Nigeria and Afghanistan are in serious state of decay.[12] Even nations that are currently making insufficient progress, such as India,[13] can accelerate maternal mortality reductions if they improve their health systems.

Motivating young people to delay pregnancy and achieve higher levels of education is best achieved through integrated community-based programmes, as well as social re-engineering to incentivise activities such as tertiary education and white collar employment, which are positively correlated with improved maternal health. In societies with high maternal mortality and morbidity, marriage is the institution through which high parity and limited educational opportunities for women occur. Thus, initiatives to delay marriage are essential for improving maternal health. A framework of intervention points for delaying childbirth is shown in Figure 13.1.

Although most nations have laws on minimum age prior to marriage, such laws are not consistently enforced. For example, although the legal age of marriage is 18 years for women and 21 for men, the actual age is much younger in most of northern India. In Jharkhand 71 per cent of Indian women married before 18 and in Uttar Pradesh 61 per cent married before age 18. In 2010, a Nigerian senator, Ahmad Sani Yerima, married a 13-year-old Egyptian girl (five years after marrying a 15-year-old Nigerian girl) and attempted to justify his actions on religious grounds. In societies where marriage represents the most feasible option for women's economic advancement, major structural drivers of gender inequality against women are likely to be operational. Social re-engineering is needed to facilitate enhanced societal prestige of formal education compared with early marriage. While marriage does not have to mean that a girl's or boy's education finishes, the attitudes of parents, schools and spouses in many societies mean that it often does. Schools often have a policy of refusing to allow married or pregnant girls or girls with babies to return. They may believe

Table 13.2 Basic compliance indicators with minimum emergency obstetric care standards

Indicator	Acceptable level
1 Availability of emergency obstetric care: basic and comprehensive care facilities	There are at least 5 emergency obstetric care facilities (including at least 1 comprehensive facility) for every 500,000 population
2 Geographical distribution of emergency obstetric care facilities	All subnational areas have at least 5 emergency obstetric care facilities (including at least 1 comprehensive facility) for every 500,000 population
3 Proportion of all births in emergency obstetric care facilities	(Minimum acceptable level to be set locally)
4 **Met need for emergency obstetric care: proportion of women with major obstetric complications who are treated in such facilities**	100% of women estimated to have major direct obstetric complication are treated in emergency obstetric care facilities
5 Caesarean sections as a proportion of all births	The estimated proportion of births by caesarean section in the population is not less than 5% or more than 15%
6 Direct obstetric case fatality rate	The case fatality rate among women with direct obstetric complications in emergency obstetric care facilities is less than 1%

Source: adapted from reference 10.

that it will set a bad example to other pupils or that other parents will be angry to see the school go against the traditional beliefs. It is therefore important to adopt a multifaceted approach to address societal perceptions to early marriage and female tertiary education.

Cameroon, a central African nation, exemplifies the impact of inadequate reproductive health services, including assisted deliveries and family planning. A summary of Cameroon's maternal health statistics is shown in Table 13.3, while Figure 13.2 depicts insufficient progress in Cameroon's achievement of MDG5's Target 5.A.

Total fertility rate in Cameroon averages five per woman. Adolescent births average 138 births per 1,000 women aged 15–19 years, compared with 17 teenage births per 1,000 women in Australia. In Cameroon, unmet need for contraception is high at 20 per cent, indicating that women may not be achieving their desired family sizes. The World Bank recommends the following approaches to improve reproductive health services in developing nations.

- Address the issue of opposition to use of contraception and promote the benefits of small family sizes. Increase family planning awareness and utilisation through outreach campaigns and messages in the media. Enlist community leaders and women's groups.
- Provide quality family planning services that include counselling and advice, focussing on young and poor populations. Highlight the effectiveness of modern contraceptive methods and properly educate women on the health risks and benefits of such methods.

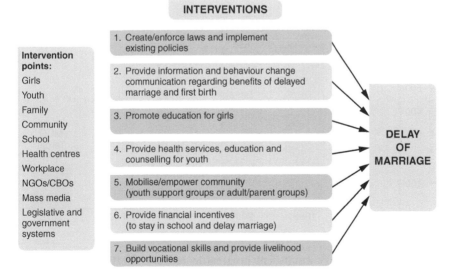

Figure 13.1 Possible pathways to delay of marriage (source: from reference 14).

Table 13.3 Cameroon's maternal mortality statistics

MDG5A indicators	
Maternal mortality ratio (maternal deaths per 100,000 live births) *UN estimate*[a]	602
Births attended by skilled health personnel (per cent)	61.8
MDG5B indicators	
Contraceptive prevalence rate (per cent)	29.2
Adolescent fertility rate (births per 1,000 women ages 15–19)	138
Antenatal care with health personnel (per cent)	83.3
Unmet need for family planning (per cent)	20.2

Source: World Bank Public Domain, reference 15.

Note
a 2004 DHS estimated MMR at 669 per 100,000 live births.

- Promote the use of all modern contraceptive methods, including long-term methods, through proper counselling which may entail training/retraining health care personnel.
- Secure reproductive health commodities and strengthen supply chain management to further increase contraceptive use as demand is generated. Promote institutional delivery through provider incentives and possibly implement risk-pooling schemes. Provide vouchers to women in hard-to-reach areas for transport and/or to cover cost of delivery services.
- Target the poor and women in hard-to-reach rural areas in the provision of basic and comprehensive emergency obstetric care (renovate and equip health facilities).

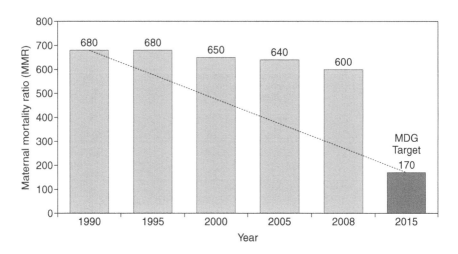

Figure 13.2 Cameroon's insufficient progress in relation to MDG5A; dotted line indicated optimal MMR reduction trend required to meet MDG target (source: World Bank Public Domain, reference 15).

- Address the inadequate human resources for health by training more midwives and deploying them to the poorest or hard-to-reach districts.
- Strengthen the referral system by instituting emergency transport, training health personnel in appropriate referral procedures (referral protocols and recording of transfers) and establishing maternity waiting huts/homes at hospitals to accommodate women from remote communities who wish to stay close to the hospital prior to delivery.
- During antenatal care, educate pregnant women about the importance of delivery with skilled health personnel and getting a postnatal check.

Cash transfers, and in particular conditional cash transfers, where households must meet certain conditions to receive the cash, have also been included in a number of programmes that have a direct or indirect focus on maternal health outcomes. The impact of conditional cash transfers on maternal health outcomes was investigated among 2006 and 2007 cohorts in El Salvador by the International Food Policy Research Institute. This study found that tying aid to maternal health programme compliance improved skilled attendance and birth in certified obstetric facilities.[16] Evidence is inconclusive about which aspect(s) of conditional cash transfers facilitate positive maternal health outcomes – the cash? The conditions? The social marketing of the programme? Nevertheless, timing is critical to engage a woman with appropriate health interventions before she gives birth, during delivery and after she gives birth.

Female health promotion programmes are essential to reduce the risks of ill health among women. In Cameroon, for example, adult HIV prevalence is 5.5 per cent, but it is 6.8 per cent among women. Reducing HIV risks among women may entail the following initiatives: integrate HIV/AIDS/STIs and family planning services in routine antenatal and postnatal care; lower the incidence of HIV infections by strengthening Behaviour Change Communication programmes via mass media and community outreach to raise HIV/AIDS awareness and knowledge.[15]

Marketing best practice interventions for reducing maternal mortality is a useful approach to diffusing innovations in this area. A 2008 World Vision document entitled *Reducing Maternal, Newborn and Child Deaths in the Asia-Pacific: Strategies that Work*[17] describes initiatives such as the Chiranjeevi safe motherhood project which funds antenatal care institutional deliveries for all pregnant women living below the poverty line in Gujarat. The scheme was well targeted, with at least 80 per cent of all poor women covered. Institutional deliveries rose from 38 per cent to 59 per cent at the end of the pilot phase. A review of maternal mortality reduction programmes in five South Asian nations revealed that removal of financial barriers to obstetric care and decentralisation of maternal health services improved service use and availability. However, the generalisability of the efficacy projects reviewed is difficult to ascertain.[18]

Capacity building for maternal mortality reduction

An interesting paradox in maternal mortality capacity building is observed in South Africa where the government spends $748 per person per year on public health, 87 per cent of deliveries take place in hospitals or under skilled health workers' supervision, yet 4,500 women die each year of pregnancy-related causes, and maternal mortality ratio increased from 150 deaths per 100,000 live births in 1998 to 625/100,000 in 2007. While HIV played a significant role in South Africa's worsening maternal mortality statistics, poor organisational capacity is also an important contributor. In a 2011 Human Rights Watch report entitled *Stop Making Excuses: Accountability for Maternal Health Care in South Africa*, a survey of 157 women in the country's poorest province, the Eastern Cape, found widespread evidence of unprofessional practices. Some women had been chastised for being pregnant, made to clean up their own blood or denied services because they were foreign. One South African woman delivered a stillborn baby after waiting for three hours to see a doctor at a district hospital; nurses had told her she was lying about being in labour.[19]

Thus, capacity building for maternal mortality needs to explore and integrate the multiple influences on this public health problem and implement sustainable interventions. At international and national levels, maternal mortality needs to be reconceptualised as a human rights issue, not just a health and development issue. Maternal health is closely aligned to a right to the highest attainable standard of health. Human rights treaty protections relevant to reducing maternal mortality are detailed in the Convention on the Elimination of All Forms of Discrimination Against Women, as well as the International Covenant on Economic, Social and Cultural Rights.[20] It is important to develop adequate capacity among civil service organisations, public health experts and human rights activists to advocate for reduction in maternal mortality as a human right rather than as a charity.

Building adequate capacity for international aid coordination for reducing maternal mortality is important. In 2008, the United Nations Fund for Population Activities established the Maternal Health Thematic Fund (MHTF) as a performance-based, MDG-driven mechanism to accelerate progress towards maternal mortality reduction in nations with highest prevalence. It plays a catalytic role in strengthening national capacities to achieve universal quality maternal health care, leverage global, national and regional awareness as well as foster national commitment and action. In 2010, the MHTF had an operating budget of US$27 million and expenditure of US$21 million. It provided assistance to 30 nations, including Afghanistan, Nigeria and Ethiopia. The MHTF programme also targets obstetric fistula prevention and rehabilitation of survivors. Examples of capacity building initiatives in relation to medical and socioeconomic rehabilitation of fistula survivors include the Livelihood Empowerment

Against Poverty programme in Ghana and mobile-to-mobile banking technology for survivors of obstetric fistula in Tanzania.[21]

At national levels, capacity building for development of quality emergency obstetric care is a priority in most nations with high maternal mortality ratios.[10] As part of capacity building activities, the following research needs and information gaps need to be addressed for specific contexts.[22]

- Studies on community perceptions of obstetric complications as determinants of women's health seeking behaviour. Results will be useful for designing *information–education–communication* messages.
- Identification of innovative techniques for community education (to raise awareness of complications, to recognise complications and the need to seek timely care) and community mobilisation (to ensure availability of transport and availability of funds).
- Identification of the most cost-effective approaches to extend obstetric care, into the community. How do we best maximise essential obstetric care coverage? (Upgrade the skills of rural physicians in emergency obstetric care? Upgrade the skills of non-physician personnel (nurse-midwives and midwives) to manage obstetric emergencies and delegate responsibility to them?)
- Research and analysis to document best practices and lessons learned in delegating responsibility for emergency obstetric care (this should include impact of responsibility delegation, lessons learned, acceptability of greater responsibility of care by non-physician health staff and physicians, and approaches used to influence national policy regarding responsibility delegation).
- In most African countries, midwives are reluctant to work in rural areas, and traditional birth attendants are the only alternative for pregnant women. There is a need to conduct local studies to determine the causes of attrition and increased turnover of trained personnel in rural areas and to identify ways of counteracting them.
- Operations research on models of first referral level facilities. Some health centres as well as rural and district hospitals have been upgraded to provide emergency obstetric care services. What has been learned so far about first referral level facilities? Evaluate first referral level facilities providing emergency obstetric care to assess their efficiency, effectiveness and impact on maternal mortality and morbidity. Identify best practices and lessons learned. Which services provided at first referral level facilities most effectively reduce maternal mortality and morbidity?
- Many women with obstetric complications die because of the inadequacy of the referral system. What factors constitute an effective referral system? What is needed for a functioning referral system? Research may be needed to reliably determine adequacy, costs and impact on maternal mortality and morbidity of different approaches used in

different settings for referral to a facility with obstetric services. What innovative strategies are likely to be required to enhance the referral system, linking providers at the community level, health centre level and hospital level to respond to obstetric complications?

- Situation analysis of efficiency and effectiveness of current strategies for provision of emergency obstetric care (includes infrastructure, human resource capacity, referral and communications network capability). The information on institutional capacity provided by the situation analysis will be useful in the development of improved protocols, guidelines and interventions.
- Research on models providing emergency obstetric care, including assessment of relative cost-effectiveness of different obstetric interventions.
- Research to identify appropriate financing and cost-recovery measures for providing emergency obstetric care services in different settings.

Capacity building for improving obstetrician and midwifery workforce, quantity, quality and distribution is high priority in most developing nations. A coalition of credible international health organisations issued a position statement on midwifery workforce capacity building in 2010 (Figure 13.3).

Capacity building for health systems improvement is essential to provide comprehensive maternal and child health services. For example, Sri Lanka reduced maternal deaths from between 550 per 100,000 live births in 1950 to 38 per 100,000 live births in 2008. The commendable decline is attributable to four major factors: broad, free access to a strong health system; the professionalisation and broad use of midwives; gathering of health information and use of this information for policy making; targeted quality improvements to vulnerable groups.

Sri Lanka accomplished its large reduction in maternal mortality while spending a smaller percentage of GDP on health than most countries at its income level. Maternal mortality decreased more rapidly than female death rates in general. Suicide rates among women in Sri Lanka remain the highest in the world (21/100,000 people), despite tremendous improvements in maternal mortality rates. This trend suggests that maternal mortality fell due to factors other than general improvements in health. Up scaling of health systems will result in greater correlation between improvements in maternal mortality and improvements in maternal health in general.

Continuing education is an effective capacity building tool for reducing maternal mortality. Such training programmes keep staff abreast of current developments in maternal health, and facilitate dissemination of best practice policies and programmes. For example, ALARM (Advances in Labour and Risk Management) International Program is a training tool developed by the Society of Obstetricians and Gynaecologists of Canada, which aims to reduce death and injury caused by pregnancy, childbirth and unsafe abortion in countries with high maternal mortality and morbidity rates. The five-day programme targets health professionals who provide obstetric care, reviewing the top maternal killers and suggesting essential tools and problem management with the goal of improving care for mothers and newborns.[23]

Capacity building for encouraging pregnant women in nations with high prevalence of maternal mortality to have in-facility deliveries is an

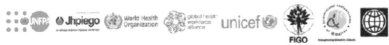

A GLOBAL CALL TO ACTION: STRENGTHEN MIDWIFERY TO SAVE LIVES AND PROMOTE HEALTH OF WOMEN AND NEWBORNS (6 June 2010)

Maternal Mortality: Still the greatest health and gender inequity in the world
We, midwives and other health professionals of the world and development partners, gathered here on the occasion of the Women Deliver Conference in Washington DC, June 2010, share the view that bold and unprecedented action is required to achieve Millennium Development Goal (MDG) 5: *Improve Maternal Health* and the newborn component of MDG4: *Reduce child mortality*. Today 99 per cent of maternal and newborn deaths occur in developing countries. Each year more than two million women and newborns die needlessly due to preventable causes related to pregnancy, childbirth and post-partum conditions. Millions more suffer disabilities. When a woman dies, her children are less likely to receive nutritious food and education. Saving women's lives and improving their health are key to achieving all of the MDGs.

We know what to do – it is a cost-effective investment
There is international consensus on the set of evidence-based and cost-effective solutions required to ensure that *every pregnancy is wanted, every birth is safe and every newborn is healthy*. Central to these interventions is a high quality workforce supported by a functioning health system. Midwives, as part of this workforce, provide the continuum of care needed by pregnant women and their newborns from the community to the hospital level.

Midwives and midwifery services save lives and promote health
Up to 90 per cent of maternal deaths can be prevented when midwives and personnel with midwifery skills are authorized and supported by the health system to practice their full set of competencies, including basic emergency obstetric and newborn care. In addition midwives improve the sexual and reproductive health of individuals and couples, including adolescents, by providing family planning services and counseling, and HIV prevention, including the prevention of mother-to-child transmission of HIV. According to the World Health Organization (WHO), some *334,000 midwives are needed* to fill the gaps in high-mortality countries by 2015.

A Call to Action to strengthen midwifery services
We pledge to join forces with governments, civil society, and other partners to continue supporting implementation of World Health Assembly Resolution 59.27 on Strengthening nursing and midwifery and initiating a global movement to strengthen midwifery services. This will ensure rapid progress in achieving MDG 5 and contribute to the achievement of MDGs 4 and 6 (to reduce child mortality; and combat HIV/AIDS, malaria, and other diseases). In response to the UN Secretary General's Joint Action Plan for Women's and Children's Health, we call on all governments to increase investments in midwifery services now and to make this a high priority at the UN Summit on the Millennium Development Goals in September 2010 and beyond.

We call on governments to address the following vital areas:

1. **Education and training**—Provide education and training in the essential competencies for basic midwifery practice. Build institutional capacity, including strengthened clinical training, post-graduate programs and research. Increase South-South collaboration to expand the production of midwives with evidence-based quality training.

2. **Legislation and Regulation**—Strengthen legislative and regulatory frameworks to ensure midwives have appropriate standards of practice and are regulated to practice their full set of competencies as defined by the WHO and the International Confederation of Midwives (ICM). Also, ensure immediate notification of maternal deaths.

3. **Recruitment, retention and deployment**—Implement national, costed health workforce plans and strengthen management capacities of Ministries of Health regarding training, recruitment, retention and deployment of the midwifery workforce, as per *The 2008 Kampala Declaration and Agenda for Global Action on Health Workers* and which is vital to increasing access to midwifery services for poor and marginalized women.

4. **Association**—Strengthen national professional midwifery associations to promote the profession, improve standards of care, participate in policy making at regional and national levels, and establish closer collaboration with other professional organizations, especially obstetric and pediatric societies.

Figure 13.3 Advocacy for improving midwifery services – Position Statement by coalition of stakeholders (source: United Nations Fund for Population Activities, (public domain) available from: www.unfpa.org/webdav/site/global/shared/documents/events/2010/midwifery/Joint_Statement_Symposium_on_Strengthening_Midwifery_Final_04JUN2010.pdf (accessed 1 April 2012)).

important approach to reducing maternal mortality. Two promising approaches are: (1) equipping and resourcing of maternity waiting rooms, coordinated with funding of transportation for pregnant women in remote regions, and (2) conditional cash transfer to facilitate adherence with antenatal care schedule, and encourage deliveries in equipped health centres. In most developing nations, maternity waiting rooms are associated with significantly improved maternal and child health outcomes, provided they are strategically located, closely linked to well-resourced delivery centres and free for use by pregnant women. Although most evaluation studies are not rigorous, the leitmotiv of reviewed studies conducted in low socioeconomic settings is that this approach significantly reduces maternal mortality. For example, the top ten causes for maternal death in a rural Ethiopia setting between 1998 and 2008, separated by usage of maternity waiting area, are shown in Table 13.4.

Building capacity for maternity waiting areas involves substantial budget for infrastructure, transport or transport subsidies, and on-call midwives and obstetricians. Economies of scale may make this option unattractive in sparsely populated regions or areas with low birth rates.

The use of conditional cash transfers to facilitate reductions in maternal mortality and improve antenatal care is best exemplified by India's Janani Suraksha Yojana (JSY) conditional cash payment scheme. Established in 2001, the JSY scheme is a conditional cash transfer to increase births in adequately resourced health centres. It is focussed on pregnant women in ten states: Uttar Pradesh, Kashmir, Orissa, Jharkhand, Bihar, Uttaranchal, Assam, Rajasthan, Jammu and Madhya Pradesh. These states have low rates of hospital/health centre deliveries. The JSY had a significant effect on completion of antenatal care and in-facility births. This scheme was associated with a reduction of 3.7 per cent (95 per cent CI:

Table 13.4 Causes of maternal death in relation to use of maternity waiting rooms in rural Ethiopia, 1998–2008

Cause	Maternity waiting area	No maternity waiting area
Postpartum haemorrhage	1	14
Hypertensive disease	0	11
Sepsis	0	5
Obstructed labour	0	18
Complicated abortion	0	4
Cerebral malaria	0	11
Severe anaemia	0	6
Cardiac disease	1	1
Relapsing fever	0	1
Total	2	71

Source: adapted from reference 24.

Table 13.5 Estimated maternal and newborn deaths averted through implementation of Chiranjeevi Yolana scheme in Gujarat, 2005–2009

Total deliveries under Chiranjeevi scheme	Expected maternal deaths	Maternal deaths reported under Chiranjeevi scheme	Mothers saved under Chiranjeevi scheme	Expected early neonatal deaths	Early neonatal deaths reported under Chiranjeevi scheme	Early neonates saved
332,151	531	62	469	7,639	1,276	6,363

Source: reference 26.

2.2–5.2) perinatal deaths per 1,000 pregnancies and 2.3 per cent (95 per cent CI: 0.97–3.7) neonatal deaths.[25] In the Indian state of Gujarat, fee waiver programmes for women who elect to deliver in hospital under the 'Chiranjeevi Yolana' programme cost US$12.6/year, or 3.6 per cent of the state's annual health budget. The programme has been credited with saving about 400 mothers and 5,300 newborns between 2005 and 2010,[26] although this estimate is not based on rigorous evaluation (Table 13.5 and Figure 13.4).

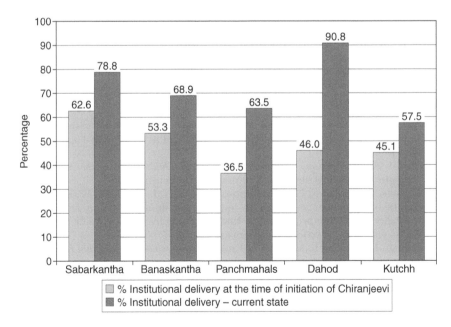

Figure 13.4 Attributed influence of Chiranjeevi Yolana scheme in Gujarat on in-hospital deliveries, selected districts, 2005–2010 (source: (public domain) available from: www.gujhealth.gov.in/Images/pdf/chiran-jeevi-report1.pdf (accessed 1 April 2012) (reference 26)).

References

1 World Health Organization. *Maternal Mortality.* Geneva: WHO, 2002.
2 Loudon, I. Maternal mortality in the past and its relevance to developing countries today. *American Journal of Clinical Nutrition,* 2000; 72: s2415–s2416.
3 Noakes, T.D., Boresen, J., Hew-Butler, T., Lambert, M.I., Jordaan, E. Semmelweis and the aetiology of puerperal sepsis 160 years on: an historical review. *Epidemiology and Infection,* 2008; 136: 1–9.
4 De Costa, C.M. 'The contagiousness of childbed fever': a short history of puerperal sepsis and its treatment. *Medical Journal of Australia,* 2002; 177: 668–671.
5 United Nations Development Programme. *Millennium Development Goals.* New York, UNDP, 2005.
6 Ronsmans, C., Graham, W.J., *Lancet* Maternal Survival Series steering group. Maternal mortality: who, when, where, and why. *Lancet,* 2006; 368: 1189–1200.
7 The World Bank. *Millennium Development Goals: Maternal Mortality.* Washington, DC: World Bank, 2008.
8 World Health Organization. *Trends in Maternal Mortality: 1990 to 2008. Estimates developed by WHO, UNICEF, UNFPA and the World Bank.* Geneva: WHO, 2010.
9 Rooks, J., Winikoff, B., Bruce, J. Technical Summary: Seminar on 'Reassessment of the concept of reproductive risk in maternity care and family planning services'. New York: The Population Council, 1990.
10 World Health Organization. *Emergency Obstetric Care: A Handbook.* Geneva: WHO, 2009.
11 Fernando, D.N. Orienting Health systems for maternal health: the Sri Lankan experience. *Development,* 2005; 48: 127–136.
12 Okumura, J. Reconstruction of health care in Afghanistan. *Lancet,* 2007; 359: 1072.
13 The World Bank. *India: Reducing Infant and Maternal Mortality in Tamil Nadu.* Washington, DC: World Bank, 2009.
14 United States Agency for International Development. *Community-based Interventions to Delay Age of Marriage: A Review of Evidence in India.* Washington, DC: Intrahealth international-USAID, 2008.
15 The World Bank. *Reproductive Health at a Glance: Cameroon.* Washington, DC: World Bank, 2011.
16 International Food Policy Research Institute. Can conditional cash transfers improve maternal health and birth outcomes? IFPRI Discussion Paper 01080, New Delhi, 2011.
17 World Vision. *Reducing Maternal, Newborn and Child Deaths in the Asia-Pacific: Strategies that Work.* Melbourne: University of Melbourne, 2008.
18 Hussein, J., Newlands, D., D'Ambruoso, L., Thaver, I., Talukder, R., Besana, G. Identifying practices and ideas to improve the implementation of maternal mortality reduction programmes: findings from five South Asian countries. *British Journal of Obstetrics and Gynaecology,* 2010; 117: 304–313.
19 Human Rights Watch. *Stop Making Excuses: Accountability for Maternal Health Care in South Africa.* New York: HRW, 2011.
20 Hunt, P., De Mesquati, B. *Reducing Maternal Mortality: The Right to the Highest Attainable Standard of Health.* Essex: UNFPA, 2009.
21 United Nations Fund for Population Activities. *Maternal Health Thematic Fund.* New York: UNFPA, 2010.
22 Post, M. Preventing maternal mortality through emergency obstetric care. SARA Issues Paper, USAID, 1997.
23 International Women's Health Program. *ALARM International Maternal Mortality Reduction Training Tool.* Ottawa: RCSOG, 2006.

24 Kelly, J., Kohls, E., Poovan, P., Schiffer, R., Redito, A., Winter, H., MacArthur, C. The role of maternity waiting area (MWA) in reducing maternal mortality and stillbirths in high-risk women in rural Ethiopia. *British Journal of Obstetrics and Gynaecology*, 2010; 117: 1377–1383.
25 Lim, S.S., Dandona, L., Hotsington, J.A., James, S.L., Hogan, M.C., Gakidou, E. India's Janani Suraksha Yojana, a conditional cash transfer programme to increase births in health facilities: an impact evaluation. *Lancet*, 2010; 375: 2009–2023.
26 Gujarat Ministry of Health and Family Welfare. Chiranjeevi Gujarat: An innovative partnership with the private sector obstetricians to provide skilled care at birth to the poor in India. Health and Family Welfare Department, Government of Gujarat, 2010.

14 Capacity building for facilitating optimal resource allocation to disease prevention and health promotion

Prevention matters

The cliché 'prevention is better than cure' is better known in words than in deeds. Since the times of Hippocrates 2,500 years ago, the environment was considered an important factor in people's health and wellbeing. Disease was thought to result when environmental influences involving air, water, food or other aspects of life and health – whether seasonal or otherwise – destabilised people's 'humoral equilibrium'. Changes in the seasons and other natural influences, as well as characteristics of climate and location, could and did give rise to diseases. The author of the Hippocratic treatise 'Airs, Waters, Places' associates seasons, prevailing winds and the quality of the air and water with the physical condition of people and the occurrence of disease. Apart from the environment, optimal nutrition was regarded as a natural disease prevention tool. 'Let food be thy medicine and medicine be thy food' is a popular Hippocratic quote.[1] Since the last 150 years, activities designed (usually with active involvement of governments) to promote health, prolong life and prevent diseases come under the categories of 'public health', 'community/social medicine' and 'population health'. Public health's primary focus is disease prevention and health promotion. In the United States, the Centers for Disease Control and Prevention's list of ten major achievements of public health entails:[2]

- Vaccination, which has resulted in the eradication of smallpox, elimination of poliomyelitis in the Americas and control of measles, rubella, tetanus, diphtheria, Haemophilus influenzae type b and other infectious diseases.
- Improvements in motor-vehicle safety have resulted from engineering efforts to make both vehicles and highways safer and from successful efforts to change personal behaviour (e.g. increased use of safety belts, child safety seats and motorcycle helmets, and decreased drinking and driving). These efforts have contributed to large reductions in motor-vehicle-related deaths.

- Work-related health problems, such as coal workers' pneumoconiosis (black lung), and silicosis – common at the beginning of the century – have come under better control. Severe injuries and deaths related to mining, manufacturing, construction and transportation also have decreased; since 1980, safer workplaces have resulted in a reduction of approximately 40 per cent in the rate of fatal occupational injuries.
- Control of infectious diseases has resulted from clean water and improved sanitation. Infections such as typhoid and cholera transmitted by contaminated water, a major cause of illness and death early in the twentieth century, have been reduced dramatically by improved sanitation. In addition, the discovery of antimicrobial therapy has been critical to successful public health efforts to control infections such as tuberculosis and sexually transmitted diseases.
- Decline in deaths from coronary heart disease and stroke have resulted from risk-factor modification, such as smoking cessation and blood pressure control coupled with improved access to early detection and better treatment. Since 1972, death rates for coronary heart disease have decreased 51 per cent.
- Since 1900, safer and healthier foods have resulted from decreases in microbial contamination and increases in nutritional content. Identifying essential micronutrients and establishing food-fortification programmes have almost eliminated major nutritional deficiency diseases such as rickets, goitre and pellagra in the United States.
- Healthier mothers and babies have resulted from better hygiene and nutrition, availability of antibiotics, greater access to health care and technologic advances in maternal and neonatal medicine. Since 1900, infant mortality has decreased 90 per cent, and maternal mortality has decreased 99 per cent.
- Access to family planning and contraceptive services has altered social and economic roles of women. Family planning has provided health benefits such as smaller family size and longer interval between the birth of children, increased opportunities for pre-conception counselling and screening, fewer infant, child and maternal deaths, and the use of barrier contraceptives to prevent pregnancy and transmission of human immunodeficiency virus and other venereal diseases.
- Fluoridation of drinking water began in 1945 and in 1999 reaches an estimated 144 million persons in the United States. Fluoridation safely and inexpensively benefits both children and adults by effectively preventing tooth decay, regardless of socioeconomic status or access to care. Fluoridation has played an important role in the reduction in tooth decay (40–70 per cent in children) and of tooth loss in adults (40–60 per cent).
- Recognition of tobacco use as a health hazard and subsequent public health anti-smoking campaigns have resulted in changes in social norms to prevent initiation of tobacco use, promote cessation of use

and reduce exposure to environmental tobacco smoke. Since the 1964 Surgeon General's report on the health risks of smoking, the prevalence of smoking among adults has decreased, and millions of smoking-related deaths have been prevented.

Prevention is not cheap, but it is generally more cost-effective curative care. However, it does not have the same level of visibility and consumer acknowledgement as hospital-based clinical care. It also usually implies a change in industrial, personal lifestyle and business practices, factors which tend to reduce its attractiveness to key stakeholders.

Sometimes public health becomes a victim of its own success, and limited foresight by government health policy makers stifles public health programmes. In Washington, United States, smoking rates dropped by one-third, from 22 per cent to 15 per cent in the decade since the Washington State Tobacco Control Program was constituted, with funding of at least $26 million annually. A 15 per cent regular smoking rate was the third lowest in the United States in 2010. Studies in other American states show that state-funded tobacco control programmes contribute significantly to reducing smoking initiation and prevalence.[3] As a result of drastic budget cuts, Washington's tobacco prevention programme now has a very small amount of funding that it uses to enforce laws against selling tobacco to minors and to help develop smoke-free policy. But there's no longer any media campaigns targeting young people and adults, or any funding for school-based efforts, and the state's Quitline, which in 2010 was getting an average of 1,900 calls a month, is no longer supported with state funds and now only serves those who can pay.

In December 2011, the Australian government decided to axe a $200 million funding designed to assist people with multiple risk factors for diabetes to be referred to a six-week course on changing their diet and activity levels to reduce their chance of getting the illness. This cut came despite two million Australian adults at risk of Type 2 diabetes and studies which had shown that the programme was successful. Diabetes Australia Policy Adviser, Professor Greg Johnson, criticised the cuts, stating:

> Diabetes is one of the major drivers of preventable hospital admissions. About one-third of preventable admissions are related to diabetes and its complications ... If we want to make inroads into the huge costs within our hospital system, we need to invest more into diabetes, not less.[4]

In the United States, a study which sought to determine whether changes in health care spending by local public health agencies impacted on rates in mortality from chronic diseases found that mortality rates fell between 1.1 per cent and 6.9 per cent for each 10 per cent increase in local public health spending directed towards child health, diabetes prevention and cancer prevention (Table 14.1).[5]

Table 14.1 Effects of local public health spending on community mortality rates

Mortality rate	% change per 10% increase in spending
Infant deaths per 1,000 live births	−6.85**
Heart disease deaths per 100,000 population	−3.22**
Diabetes deaths per 100,000 population	−1.44**
Influenza deaths per 100,000 population	−1.13**
All-cause deaths per 100,000 population	−0.25**

Source: adapted from reference 5.

Notes
**$P < 0.05$.

The 2011 Cancer Research UK Report stated that 40 per cent of cancers are preventable through addressing modifiable lifestyle risks such as smoking, alcohol, obesity and inadequate intake of fruits and vegetables. Tobacco remains the most avoidable cause of cancer, responsible for at least 20 per cent of cases. Addressing these cancer pathways through prevention programmes contributed significantly to halving the probability of death before the age of 70 in the UK over the last 35 years.[6]

Most studies indicate the large benefits of public health spending in order to improve population health and to reduce costs of clinical services. However, in most countries, public health funding budget is minuscule not only in real terms, but also in relation to spending in other health sector. In Australia as at 2009/2010, government devoted 1.7 per cent of total budget of $116.3 billion to public health and 5 per cent to community health. Spending on public health in Australia declined by 13.7 per cent, in real terms, between 1999 and 2009.[7] Similar trends have been noted in most other nations. Capacity building is a potentially useful approach to facilitate optimal public health spending. Two important areas for intervention are *advocacy* and *legislation*.

Advocacy for optimal public health funding

The roots of advocacy may be traced to the 5 BC Hippocratic teachings entitled 'On Airs Water and Places', in which it was stated:

> Whoever wishes to investigate medicine properly should … consider … the mode in which inhabitants live, and what are their pursuits, whether they are fond of drinking and eating to excess, and given to indolence, or are fond of exercise and labour.[1]

Although he was primarily focussed in encouraging doctors to be patient advocates, healers of the Hippocratic era were cognisant of the importance of environmental and lifestyle factors in disease causation. Lifestyle factors are thought to account for 40 per cent of cancers, while the following environmental factors have been linked to rising cancer prevalence globally:[8]

- *metals* such as arsenic and cancers of the bladder, lung and skin;
- *chlorination byproducts* such as trihalomethanes and bladder cancer;
- *natural fibres* such as asbestos and cancers of the larynx, lung, mesothelioma and stomach;
- *petrochemicals and combustion products*, including motor vehicle exhaust and polycyclic aromatic hydrocarbons, and cancers of the bladder, lung and skin.
- *pesticide* exposures and cancers of the brain, wilms tumour, leukaemia and non-Hodgkin's lymphoma;
- *reactive chemicals* such as vinyl chloride and liver cancer and soft tissue sarcoma;
- *metalworking fluids and mineral oils* with cancers of the bladder, larynx, nasal passages, rectum, skin and stomach;
- *ionising radiation* and cancers of the bladder, bone, brain, breast, liver, lung, ovary, skin and thyroid, as well as leukaemia, multiple myeloma and sarcomas;
- *solvents* such as benzene and leukaemia and non-Hodgkin's lymphoma, tetrachloroethylene and bladder cancer, and trichloroethylene and Hodgkin's disease, leukaemia, and kidney and liver cancers.

Advocating for improved public protection from environmental carcinogens rests on research evidence (i.e. 'precision') as well as public awareness campaigns and lobbying governments to institute environmental protection policies. Advocates armed with adequate facts are better able to frame health policy questions in a manner that would accord it high priority.

Edwin Chadwick, lawyer and sanitary reformer, heralded the modern era of public health advocacy. His chief contribution was his unrelenting campaign for entrusting certain departments of local affairs to trained and selected experts, instead of to representatives elected on the principle of local self-government. His report on 'The Sanitary Condition of the Labouring Population' (~1842) remains a valuable historical document. His advocacy mantra was 'all miasma is disease'. Although technically wrong, this advocacy effort resulted in major improvements in sanitation, a centralised sewerage system for England and Wales, and culminated in the promulgation of the world's first Public Health Act in 1848.[9] Unlike Chadwick, who advocated from a Functionalist perspective, Marx and Engels were Structuralists, more focussed on addressing the socioeconomic and political underpinnings of health inequality. For example, in their respective publications examining the health conditions of the working classes in England, Chadwick and Engels identified basically the same set of adverse public health factors. However, while Chadwick sought to address the adverse health issues without disrupting the existing socio-political system, Engels sought to radically reform society's social structures to achieve the same ends.[10] These two historical figures demonstrated two advocacy approaches to secure adequate funding for public health. A simple description of 'advocacy' is that it is the act of pleading for, supporting or recommending a course of action. However, such a description does not adequately distinguish advocacy from related activities such as public education or social marketing.

'Advocacy' is derived from the Latin/Italian term 'Avvocati', meaning 'one who argues on behalf of himself or others, especially for fair, equal or/and humane treatment'. In law, advocacy is a key function of barristers. Advocacy is used in a number of contexts in health, e.g. self-advocacy, group advocacy, policy advocacy, media advocacy and public health advocacy. As briefly discussed in Chapter 6, public health advocacy seeks to bridge the gap between what is being done and what needs to be done to speed progress in reducing diseases or injuries. It does this by placing and keeping public health issues firmly on the public and political agenda, shaping debate about public health issues, addressing barriers to the adoption of policies or adequate funding of programmes and countering the activities of interest groups intended to undermine support for change. Methods and avenues used by public health advocates include civil disobedience, exposure of industry conduct and lobbyists, media advocacy, counter-advertising, political lobbying, mobilisation of community groups, recruitment of respected champions, strategic use of research, public meetings or events, personal and professional networks, petitions and newsletters, Internet-based advocacy technologies.

A standard definition of public health advocacy is provided by the author: 'Process of surmounting or sidestepping ideological obstacles that impair conditions for healthy living. Effective public health advocates use the right mix of the 5ps – Precision, Passion, Promptitude, Perseverance, and Personality – to facilitate improvements in public health.'[11] Racism is an advocacy issue with significant adverse health and community-wide implications.[12] The late Martin Luther King Jr (MLK) was a pre-eminent anti-racism advocate who skilfully applied the '5 Ps' of public health advocacy. In relation to 'precision', he used the prosecution of Mary Parks for sitting in a whites-only section of Alabama's public buses to institute a legal challenge against race-based segregation in public transport in Montgomery, Alabama, and at the same time organised a mass boycott of Montgomery's public transport system by African Americans in 1955. His advocacy led to the annulment of race-based discrimination in all public transport in the United States by 1957. MLK was an erudite orator. His passion for his advocacy topic of racism is exemplified by his 'I have a dream' speech of 1963, arguably the most memorable speech of the twentieth century. Promptitude in relation to this speech is exemplified by it being delivered in the grounds of Abraham Lincoln memorial – the American president who waged a war against Southern separatists and slave owners. MLK's 'dream' speech, delivered in 1963, on the steps of the Lincoln Memorial, was 100 years after the signing of the 13th and 14th amendments. MLK's perseverance is exemplified by the fact that he suffered scores of arrests and several imprisonments, mainly on trumped-up charges. Eventually, he was assassinated in 1968 in Memphis, Tennessee at the age of 39. MLK's towering personality was a major asset in his advocacy efforts. He was a peaceful warrior, prominent, pre-eminent and difficult to ignore.

Contemporary uses of advocacy include efforts to convince religious and opinion leaders in northern Nigeria that polio vaccination is safe;[13] and advocacy against pharmaceutical giant Pfizer, who conducted a trial using the unlicensed drug Trovafloxacin for treating 100 Nigerian children against cerebrospinal meningitis in 1996. Claims by Pfizer that approval was given by the Kano general hospital were denied by hospital authorities. Parents claimed that they did not provide informed consent. In 2011, following adverse publicity by advocacy groups such as Centre for Research on Multinational Corporations, Pfizer made an out-of-court settlement of US$75 million, comprising $35 million to compensate the families of children in the study, $30 million to support health care initiatives in Kano and $10 million in legal costs.[14] Advocacy for optimal public health funding is usually undertaken via public health NGOs, disease-specific pressure groups like 'Action Against Smoking' and labour unions such as the American Public Health Association. It is an important component for capacity building and sensitisation of stakeholders to stimulate action in addressing health system constraints.

Despite its potential usefulness, advocacy is a difficult and technically demanding strategy for generating support for funding optimality in public health arena, as most funding decisions operate in a zero-sum game fashion, with losers likely in other sectors if public health funding is increased. Advocacy entails innovation, and innovation is not without his perils, as Niccolo Machiavelli reminds us in *The Prince* (1513):

> There is nothing more difficult, more perilous to conduct, nor more uncertain in its success, than to take the lead in a new order of things. The innovator has for enemies all those who have done well under the old conditions and lukewarm supporters in those who may do well under the new. This coolness arises partly from fear of the opponents who have the law on their side and partly from the incredulity of men who do not readily believe in new things until they have experience of them.[15]

Indeed, Edwin Chadwick, public health's pioneering advocate, soon discovered the perils of advocacy when his adversaries engineered his premature retirement from public service. His parting words in parliament illustrate his anger:

> The parliamentary agents are our sworn enemies, because we have reduced expenses, and consequently their fees, within reasonable limits.... The College of Physicians, and all its dependencies, because of our independent action and singular success in dealing with the cholera, when we have proved that many a Poor Law medical officer knew more than all the flash and fashionable doctors of London. All the Boards of Guardians, for we exposed their selfishness, their cruelty, their reluctance to meet and relieve the suffering poor, in the days of epidemic.[16]

Tactics used by opponents of public health advocates such as tobacco companies include public relations, third party support, sponsorship of research, expert opinion, political lobbying and electoral activities, mass media advertising, use of front groups and intermediaries, litigation, quashing access or release of data, withholding of funding, denigration of critics. Advocacy strategies are more likely to be used successfully for public health purposes in democratic nations where civil society groups and professional associations exert powerful influence on public policy. Ironically, advocacy is most needed in theocratic and kakistocratic nations like Swaziland and Myanmar. Capacity building for advocacy thus needs to address the above encumbrances. In the United States, the Prevention Institute exemplifies the impact of advocacy as a tool for securing optimal public health funding. I met executive members of this public health advocacy group at an international public health conference in Istanbul in 2009. The Prevention Institute is adequately staffed by tertiary qualified staff, most of whom work part time or on voluntary basis. They are able to source adequate funding from public and private sources. These qualities exemplify impressive capacity building efforts. On 9 December 2011, the Institute developed a public awareness message on the House Republicans' payroll tax plan which aims to increase doctors' Medicare reimbursement by dramatically cutting the Prevention and Public Health Fund by more than two-thirds. The Institute opened an online letter-signing initiative to put pressure on Congress members against cuts to the public health budget. The letter reads:[17]

> Dear Congressperson,
> The Prevention and Public Health Fund represents an unprecedented investment in public health and wellness, and is essential to ensuring the health and vitality of our communities and that of our nation. As Congress contemplates how to address the funding shortfall for Medicare reimbursements under the Sustainable Growth Rate (SGR) formula, we are dismayed to learn that the Fund is currently being

considered as a potential offset for this looming cut to Medicare providers. We urge you to reject calls to use any portion of the Fund to address the 'doc fix.'

We must address the rates that Medicare pays doctors, but doing so by raiding the prevention fund is a short-sighted solution that will cost money, not save it. Every dollar we divert from prevention will cost us as much as five dollars down the road. By reducing expenditures and reducing need in the first place, investments in comprehensive prevention bend the cost curve and stem the rising tide of expenditures on preventable chronic diseases. Quality, affordable medical care and community prevention work hand-in-hand.

By supporting local communities through $15 billion over the next ten years, the Fund advances our nation beyond a focus on sickness and treatment to one of ensuring health and well-being through innovative, evidence-based community prevention. Communities are already putting these strategies to work in their neighborhoods, addressing the chronic diseases that place the heaviest cost burdens on our health care system.

In times of great economic need, our businesses, our communities and our health care system will all benefit from more prevention funding – not cuts.

Public health is not separate from health care delivery. In fact, in a new national survey from the Robert Wood Johnson Foundation, 3 out of 4 physicians surveyed wished our current health care system would cover the costs of addressing their patients' social needs, the very needs community prevention resolves – such as lack of safe open spaces for physical activity and lack of meaningful access to affordable housing and nutritious food. Furthermore, 85% of physicians reported that it was as important to address these unmet social needs as medical conditions. Using the Fund as an offset for the 'doc fix' takes our country backward, stifling the opportunity to build a health care system where public health and health care are fully integrated. We will better advance the health and well-being of our nation by helping public health and health care work together better, not by pitting them against each other.

Sincerely,
Larry Cohen, MSW
Executive Director

Legislation as a public health tool

King Hammurabi of Babylon is credited with developing the first legal code to regulate health care practice. Codex Hammurabi was inscribed in a huge stone stele around 1700 BC, and included the following:[18]

- rates set for general surgery, eye surgery, setting fractures, curing diseased muscles and other specific health care services;
- fees set according to a sliding scale based on ability to pay;
- owners to pay for health care for their slaves;
- objective outcome measurement standards to assure quality of care;
- outcomes information management to include data collection and evaluation;
- consumer and patient's rights to be publicised, explained and made known to all.

Modern health care legislation is focussed on three main areas: laws that establish the structure, function and authority of government public health agencies at the federal, state and local government levels; laws designed to achieve specific health objectives, such as taxing tobacco products and requiring immunisation for school entry; legislation in other areas of government, such as education, transportation, land use planning and agriculture, that have health effects. In this regard, non-health sectors can contribute significantly to health by considering the health implications of their policies. For example, REACH is a regulation of the European Union, adopted to improve the protection of human health and the environment from the risks that can be posed by chemicals, while enhancing the competitiveness of the EU chemicals industry. It also promotes alternative methods for the hazard assessment of substances in order to reduce the number of tests on animals.[19]

Legislation is foundational to public health practice. Laws delineate the scope of public health agencies, authorise or delimit public health functions and appropriate essential funds.[20]

It is generally agreed that public health funding is inadequate relative to need. The Organisation for Economic Co-operation and Development (OECD) countries allocate over 90 per cent of public expenditure on health to clinical and curative health care. Investment in health promotion and disease prevention amounts, on average, to 3.1 per cent of public expenditure on health: ranging between 0.7 per cent in Iceland and 6.6 per cent in Canada. The Nairobi Call to Action, adopted in 2009 by the participants of the Seventh Global Conference on Health Promotion, promoted this model by urging countries to 'secure adequate financing by establishing stable and sustainable financing at all levels, for example health promotion foundations'.[21]

A controversial method to secure optimum funding for public health activities is the institution of a ring-fenced funding legislation, whereby funding for specified projects are insulated from spending cuts or competition. In Western Australia, the Healthway project is an example in which government legislation is utilised to earmark a proportion of tobacco taxes for general health promotion projects. Healthway (the Western Australian Health Promotion Foundation) was established in 1991 under Section 15

of the Tobacco Control Act 1990 as an independent statutory body reporting to the Minister for Health. Healthway now functions under Part 5 of
the Tobacco Products Control Act 2. The key priorities for Healthway are
reducing harm from tobacco, reducing harm from alcohol, reducing
obesity and promoting good mental health. If Healthway is successful, and
significantly reduces the consumption of tobacco products in Western
Australia, then the funds available to Healthway will be reduced. There is
some evidence that Healthway is contributing to tobacco smoking reduction in Western Australia. Of the 5,710 respondents surveyed following
Healthway sponsored health promotion events, 67 per cent were aware of
the promoted health message and 82 per cent of these understood what
the message meant. Four per cent of all respondents intended to take
action ranging from seeking information to adopting the health behaviour.[22] Smoking prevalence and uptake in Western Australia have in fact
declined steadily since the establishment of Healthway. However, it is
debatable the extent to which Healthway's activities contributed to the
decline. An alternative legislative approach to achieve the goal of s.3 of
the Tobacco Control Act, of decreasing smoking levels include subsidising
the purchase of products aimed at assisting people to quit. Critics argue
that earmarking introduces clear restrictions and inefficiencies on public
finance and reduces flexibility in the context of changing circumstances,
resulting in cutbacks in other high priority sectors. Numerous examples
demonstrate earmarked funds were used for other purposes, especially in
poor governance settings. Earmarked taxes on harmful products have
high potential in mobilising and sustaining resources to health, although
they require strong political leadership and social consensus. Amounts
generated, even if they are small, can play catalytic roles towards active
health promotion.[23]

Another approach to securing public health funding through legislation is the approach adopted in funding the Austrian Health Promotion
Foundation using a legislatively determined budget of €7.25 million annually. However, due to an average inflation rate of 2 per cent, this amount
has depreciated by 20 per cent between 1998 and 2008. Demanding a
budget increase has been delicate in Austria, partly because available
funds were not utilised. Paradoxically, it seems that the reason was not a
lack of need but a lack of institutional and public health workforce
capacity.[24]

Legislation is useful as a tool for improving public health funding and
services only if adequate capacity exists to actualise such legislation. In
the United States, for example, many local public health officials do not
have access to the legal assistance they need to address the various legal
questions that confront them. This deficit makes it harder for them to
meet their day-to-day responsibilities and makes it much more difficult
for them to use the law proactively as a method to improve public health
in their communities. In addition, many of the attorneys who provide

legal support to public health departments do not have the time or resources to develop a thorough and up-to-date understanding of public health law.[25]

India, which was badly affected by the 1994 plague outbreak in Surat has, in the past several years taken steps to implement the basic framework of the 2005 International Health Regulations (IHR), which came into effect in 2007. The requirements that need to be fulfilled by WHO member countries to comply with the IHR (2005) include: (i) designating a national IHR focal point; (ii) strengthening core capacity to detect, report and respond rapidly to public health events; (iii) assessing events that may constitute a PHEIC within 48 hours and notifying WHO within 24 hours of assessment; (iv) providing routine inspection and control activities at international airports, ports and some ground crossings; (v) examining national laws, revising health documents/forms and certificates, and building a legal and administrative framework in line with the IHR requirements. Member countries were required to complete the assessment of existing national structures and resources by June 2009, and to develop the necessary public health infrastructure and human resources to meet the IHR requirements by 2012. Challenges faced by India in implementing IHR regulations include wide variability of public health capacity in individual states and substantial financial resources to fully implement IHR principles and practices.[26]

References

1 Hippocrates. *On Airs, Waters, and Places.* University of Adelaide, 2009, translated by Adams A. ebooks@Adelaide. Available from: http://ebooks.adelaide.edu.au/h/hippocrates/airs/ (accessed 2 January 2012).

2 Centers for Disease Control. Ten great public health achievements: United States, 1900–1999. *Morbidity and Mortality Weekly Report,* 1999; 48: 291–293.

3 Farelly, C., Peachacek, T.F., Thomas, K.Y., Nelson, D. The impact of tobacco control programs on adult smoking. *American Journal of Public Health,* 2008; 98: 304–309.

4 Medew, J. $200m diabetes scheme ditched. *Sydney Morning Herald,* 19 December 2011.

5 Mays, G.P., Smith, S.A. Evidence links increases in public health spending to declines in preventable deaths. *Health Affairs,* 2011; 30: 1585–1593.

6 Peto, R. The fraction of cancer attributable to lifestyle and environmental factors in the UK in 2010. *British Journal of Cancer,* 2011; 105: S1–S1.

7 Australian Institute of Health and Welfare. *Health Expenditure Australia, 2009–2010.* Canberra: AIHW, 2010.

8 International Agency for Research on Cancer. *World Cancer Report 2008.* Lyon: IARC, 2008.

9 Hanley, J. Edwin Chadwick and the poverty of statistics. *Medical History,* 2002; 46: 21–40.

10 Engels, F. *The Condition of the Working Classes in England.* Leipzig, 1845.

11 Awofeso, N. Prison health advocacy and its changing boundaries. *International Journal of Prisoner Health,* 2008; 4: 175–183.

12 Mckenzie, K. Racism and health. *British Medical Journal,* 2003; 326: 65–66.

13 Yahya, M. Polio vaccines: 'no thank you!' barriers to polio eradication in Northern Nigeria. *African Affairs*, 2007; 106: 185–204.
14 Lenzer, J. Pfizer settles with victims of Nigerian drug trial. *British Medical Journal*, 2011; 343: d5268.
15 Waskey, A.J. *Niccolò Machiavelli: The Prince*. Milestone Documents. Available from www.milestonedocuments.com/documents/view/niccolo-machiavellis-the-prince (accessed 1 April 2012).
16 Rosen, G. *A History of Public Health*. New York: MD Publications Inc., 1958.
17 Prevention Institute. *Health Reform Advocacy*. Oakland, CA: Prevention Institute, 2011. Available from: www.preventioninstitute.org/focus-areas/reforming-our-health-system/what-you-can-do-health-reform-advocacy.html (accessed 13 December 2011).
18 Halwani, T.M., Takrouri, M.S.M. Medical laws and ethics of Babylon as read in Hammurabi's code (History). *Internet Journal of Law, Healthcare and Ethics*, 2007; 4(2).
19 European Chemicals Agency. Regulation No. 1907/2006 of the European Parliament and of the Council of 18 December 2006 concerning the Registration, Evaluation, Authorisation and Restriction of Chemicals (REACH), 2006.
20 Institute of Medicine. *For the Public's Health: Revitalising Law and Policy to meet New Challenges*. Washington, DC: National Academies of Science, 2011.
21 World Health Organization. Global Conference on Health Promotion Promoting Health and Development: Closing the Implementation Gap, 26–30 October 2009, Nairobi, Kenya.
22 Holman, C.D.J., Donovan, R.J., Corti, B., Jalleh, G., Frizzell, S.K., Carroll, A. Evaluating projects funded by the Western Australian Health Promotion Foundation: first results. *Health Promotion International*, 1996; 11: 75–88.
23 Prakongsai, P., Patcharanarumol, W., Tangcharoensathien, V. Can earmarking mobilize and sustain resources to the health sector? *Bulletin of World Health Organization*, 2008; 86(11): 898–901.
24 Schang, L.K., Czabanowska, K.M., Lin, V. Securing funds for health promotion: lessons from health promotion foundations based on experiences from Austria, Australia, Germany, Hungary and Switzerland. *Health Promotion International*, 2011; doi: 10.1093/heapro/dar023.
25 Hoffmann, D.E., Rowthorn, V. Building public health law capacity at the local level. *Journal of Law and Medical Ethics*, 2008; 36: 6–28.
26 Narain, J.P., Lal, S., Garg, R. Implementing the revised international health regulations in India. *National Medical Journal of India*, 2007; 20: 221–222.

15 Capacity building for public health emergency preparedness

Public health disasters in history

In 2010, scientists surmised that the ten plagues documented in the Old Testament book of Exodus, which devastated Egypt 3,500 years ago actually happened, and were very likely due to climate change and volcanic eruption. Archaeological evidence for these natural disasters were found in the relics of the city of Pi-Rameses on the Nile Delta, which was the capital of Egypt during the reign of Pharaoh Rameses the Second, who ruled between 1279 BC and 1213 BC. The city lay abandoned for 3,000 years, and it is speculated that plagues may have been the result. This natural disaster contributed to the decline of the ancient Egyptian empire. Modern day disasters are usually due to a combination of human and nature-related factors. Hurricane Katrina, one of the most destructive storms in the United States, struck New Orleans, Louisiana, in 2005, after canal levees broke, leaving 80 per cent of the city flooded. The limited efforts devoted to reinforcing New Orleans' storm levees, and poor social infrastructure in the most affected areas contributed to the severity of the destruction experienced.[1]

More than 350 miles of levees serve to protect New Orleans, which is mainly below sea level. On 27 August 2005, two days prior to landfall, residents were asked to evacuate, but the infrastructure to facilitate such evacuation in New Orleans was very inadequate. Most residents were poor, illiterate and one-third did not have private transport. The storm claimed at least 1,836 lives and led to losses totalling at least $100 billion.[2] The severe effects of the storm on New Orleans could not be addressed adequately to date. By 2010, the population has fallen by 60–70 per cent compared with the pre-Katrina level of 1.3 million. Many houses are left uninhabitable and derelict.[1]

The 2004 Boxing Day tsunami which struck Indonesia, Thailand, Maldives, Sri Lanka, India and the horn of Africa was caused by a magnitude 9.2 earthquake within the Indian Ocean. Striking with waves up to 30 metres high, the tsunami killed 230,000 people in 14 countries. It caused the entire planet to vibrate as much as 1 cm and triggered other earthquakes as far away as Alaska. The international community donated more than $14 billion in humanitarian aid to assist victims' families, governments of affected nations and survivors.[2]

On 26 April 1986, a catastrophic nuclear accident in Chernobyl, Ukraine, precipitated the greatest radioactive fallout in human history. Although the nuclear facility was located in Ukraine, most of the effects of radiation poisoning were reported in neighbouring Belarus, just four miles from the location of the nuclear reactor. The total release of radioactive substances was estimated at 50 million curies. This is 2,500 times that of the Windscale nuclear plant accident in England in 1957, and 16 million times that of the Three Mile Island incident in Pennsylvania in 1978. Nearly 30 radioactive isotopes had erupted from the burning reactor. Most of them were short lived, like iodine-131, tellurium-132, zirconium-95 or cerium-141. The governments of Belarus and the Soviet Union not only didn't provide the people with the necessary instructions for protection, but even made the people take part in the 1 May (Labour Day) demonstrations, thus exposing themselves to lethal radioactive isotopes. The chromosome mutations in the case of Chernobyl were mostly recessive, which means that their accumulative effect will not be obvious for several generations. However, there have been a few cases of mutation in newly born children. Cancer such as childhood leukaemia and neuroblastoma are on the rise in all areas affected by the radiation, with some isotopes such as caesium-137, strontium-90 and plutonium-239 with half-lives of 30, 29 and 24,400 years, respectively.[3]

Violence and terrorism are increasingly contributing to disasters and emergencies globally. In Pakistan, for example, 3,021 deaths occurred in terrorist attacks in 2009, up 48 per cent on the figures for 2008. A total of 12,600 deaths were attributed to violence, 14 times more than in 2006. In Iraq, 4,500 civilians were killed in 2009.[4] The most spectacular act of violence so far in the twenty-first century took place on 11 September 2001 in the United States, when Al Qaeda militants transformed passenger jets into missiles, bombing the World Trade Center and the Pentagon. The attack killed 2,753 people within hours of its occurrence, and killed thousands more from physical, toxic and psychological injuries afterwards (Figure 15.1).

For example, significant mortality increases were documented for non-rescue and non-recovery residents with intermediate exposure (adjusted hazard ratio 1.22, 95 per cent CI: 1.04–1.48).[5] The 9/11 attacks created the circumstances for the increase in violence and terrorism in Iraq, Afghanistan and Pakistan, in the context of the so-called 'war on terror'. Indeed, efforts to confront terrorism through military means, while essential, inevitably lead to public health disasters. In Sri Lanka, after several decades of terrorist activity by the Liberation Tigers of Tamil Eelam (LTTE), the Sri Lankan government under the leadership of President Rajapaksa launched a full scale war on the Tamil Tiger militants, and scored a resounding victory in May 2009. However this victory came at a great cost in military and civilian morbidity and mortality, social cohesion and infrastructure. For example, in its 2011 report on the fate of Tamil women in northern Sri Lanka, the International Crisis Group documented that 30 years of civil war between the government and LTTE has resulted in tens of thousands of female-headed households in the north and east. Families throughout those areas experienced many waves of conflict, displacement and militarisation. In the war's final stages in 2008 and 2009, hundreds of thousands of civilians in the northern Vanni region endured serial displacements and months of being shelled by the government and held hostage by the LTTE, after which they were herded into closed government camps. Most lost nearly all possessions and multiple family members, many of whom are still missing or detained as suspected LTTE cadres. When families eventually returned to villages, homes and land had been destroyed or taken over by the military. There have been alarming incidents of gender-based violence, including domestic violence within the Tamil community, in part fuelled by rising alcohol use by men. Many women have been forced into prostitution or coercive sexual relationships. Some have also been trafficked within the country and abroad.

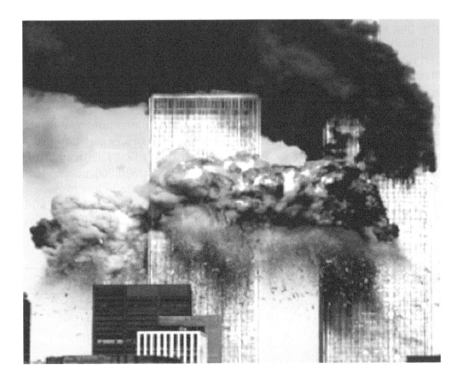

Figure 15.1 The 11 September 2001 attacks on the World Trade Center (source: photo credit: Reuters (public domain)).

Pregnancies among teenagers have increased. Fear of abuse has further restricted women's movement and impinged on education and employment opportunities.[6]

Famine, drought and food insecurity have traditionally been major contributors to disaster situations throughout human history. Despite improved food production technology, famine remains a fact of life in many parts of the developing world. The spectrum of food insecurity – as per the integrated food security phase classification (IPC) – are summarised in Table 15.1.

At a period in which obesity has become a major public health issue, two regions of the world which chronically experience major food insecurity-related humanitarian crises are North Korea and the horn of Africa. North Koreans have been experiencing prolonged food deprivation since the devastating famine of 1996–1998 killed an estimated one million citizens.[7] Despite modest improvements in harvest, North Korea faced a food deficit of at least 400,000 tons as at 2011. The death of North Korea's president Kim Jong II in December 2011 is expected to facilitate integration of this isolated and militarily repressed communist nation into the global mainstream.

Ethiopia, in the horn of Africa epitomises the disaster caused by famine, following the 1985 Live Aid concert which raised millions of dollars to assist Ethiopian famine victims. Since July 2011, a severe drought has been affecting the entire East Africa region, the worst in 60 years (Figure 15.2).

The drought has caused a severe food crisis across Somalia, Ethiopia and Kenya that threatens the livelihood of more than 13.3 million people. Many refugees from southern Somalia have fled to neighbouring Kenya and Ethiopia, where crowded, unsanitary conditions together with severe malnutrition have led to a large number of deaths.[8]

The 12 January 2010 earthquake in Haiti was a catastrophic magnitude 7.0 seismic event, with an epicentre near the town of Léogâne, approximately 25 km west of Port au Prince, Haiti's capital. By 24 January 2010, the Haitian government reported that an estimated 316,000 people had died, 300,000 had been injured and 1,000,000 made homeless. Amongst the widespread devastation and damage throughout Port au Prince and elsewhere, vital infrastructure necessary to respond to the disaster was

Table 15.1 Spectrum of food insecurity

Integrated food security phase classification	*Measurement indicators*
Generally food secure	Crude mortality rate
Chronically food insecure	Malnutrition prevalence
Acute food and livelihood crisis	Food access and availability
Humanitarian emergency	Dietary diversity
Famine/humanitarian catastrophe	Water access and availability
	Coping strategies
	Livelihood assets

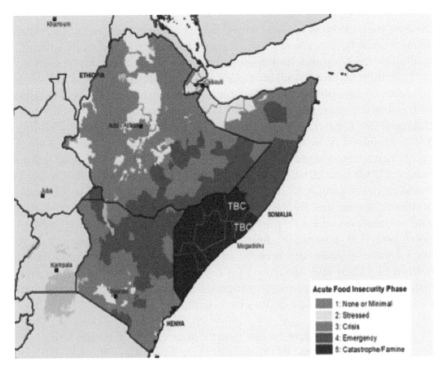

Figure 15.2 The 2011 famine in the horn of Africa (source: Wikipedia (public domain), available from: http://en.wikipedia.org/wiki/2011_East_Africa_ drought (accessed 1 April 2012)).

severely damaged or destroyed. This included all hospitals in the capital; air, sea and land transport facilities; and communication systems. Complicating this disaster, an outbreak of cholera was confirmed in Haiti on 21 October 2010, the first in 80 years. The epidemic was linked to (Nepalese) UN peacekeepers.[9] As at December 2010, 500,000 cases and 7,000 deaths have occurred as a result of the cholera epidemic, which is gradually evolving into an endemic problem in Haiti.

The humanitarian disasters discussed above exemplify the magnitude and health-related ramifications of disasters in contemporary society. While many major disasters tend to be unpredictable, health consequences are usually the most important indicators of severity and human impact. The physical, environmental and mental health consequences of disasters exert a major toll on individual well-being, community cohesion and international relations. For example, the sequence of environmental exposures after the September 2001 attacks on the World Trade Center ranged from fire, smoke, gases to particulates, all of which worsened the psychological and physical trauma of the attacks.[10]

Capacity building for emergency preparedness

Disaster preparedness is essentially a risk management process. Risk management may be described a logical and systematic method of identifying, analysing, treating and monitoring the risks involved in any activity or process, thereby using available resources efficiently. It entails establishing the context, identifying the risks, analysing the risks, evaluating the risks, addressing the risks, monitoring and review, and communication. Climate change-related emergency preparedness exemplifies capacity building efforts required of health systems. Economic losses from meteorological events have risen sevenfold from the 1960s, to an estimated US$800 billion between 2000 and 2010. Two-thirds of the economic losses are concentrated in developing nations. However, developed nations bear the brunt of deaths, disease and disability from such events. While most hazards that lead to disasters cannot be prevented, it is the ways in which societies have developed that potentiate their disaster-causing effects. Disasters have been known to erase the benefits of Millennium Development Goals in nations like Haiti and Afghanistan. Climate change has been closely associated with most modern meteorological disasters. The Inter-governmental Panel on Climate Change defines climate change as:

> a change in the state of the climate that can be identified (e.g., by using statistical tests) by changes in the mean and/or the variability of its properties, and that persists for an extended period, typically decades or longer. Climate change may be due to natural internal processes or external forces, or to persistent anthropogenic changes in the composition of the atmosphere or in land use.[11]

Thus, capacity building for disaster management should be accorded high priority by health systems. Such capacity building entails risk reduction and adaptation strategies (Figure 15.3).

Adaptation to climate change entails adjustments in natural or human systems in response to adverse climatic conditions such as flooding and drought in a matter that moderates harm or exploits beneficial opportunities. Climate change mitigation entails human intervention to reduce the sources or enhance the sinks of greenhouse gases. Examples include using fossil fuels more efficiently for industrial processes or electricity generation, switching to renewable energy (solar energy or wind power), improving the insulation of buildings and expanding forests and other 'sinks' to remove greater amounts of carbon dioxide from the atmosphere. Disaster risk reduction refers to the practice of reducing disaster risks through systematic efforts to analyse and manage the causal factors of disasters, including through reduced exposure to hazards, lessened vulnerability of people and property, wise management of land and the environment, and improved preparedness for adverse events.

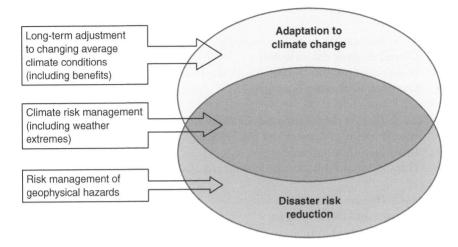

Figure 15.3 Climate change adaptation and risk reduction (adapted from reference 12).

The bulk of meteorological disasters in the first decade of the twenty-first century occurred in Asian nations. Capacity building for preventing climate change-related disasters entails learning and various types of training, but also continuous efforts to develop institutions, political awareness, financial resources, technology systems, and the wider social and cultural enabling environment. The Asian Disaster Preparedness Center (ADPC) is one such remarkable regional capacity building initiative. ADPC supports disaster-related activities within a disaster risk management framework.[13] Such a framework is based on a risk management national policy, and monitored for results through interlocking, accountable coordinating committees and implementing agencies at national, intermediate and local levels. Training in emergency preparedness and response is an important capacity tool. For example, the forty-first ADPC regional disaster management training course was held in Bangkok in February 2012.[14] The objectives of the course were to:

- identify and assess disaster risks using a risk management approach;
- plan and develop effective strategies and systems for disaster risk reduction;
- develop effective processes for preparedness planning in order to improve disaster response and recovery activities;
- effectively and efficiently set up and utilise an emergency coordination centre to manage disaster events;
- address and assess key implementation issues and requirements in disaster management.

Conducted over a period of three weeks, the course is divided into seven modules following the flow of the disaster management process.

Module 1: Introduction to disaster management
- Global disaster risk situation;
- Basic concepts and terminologies used in disaster management;
- Overview of disaster management.

Module 2: Disaster risk identification and assessment
- Introduction to disaster risk management processes;
- Introduction to hazards;
- Hazard, vulnerability, capacity and risk assessment.

Module 3: Disaster risk reduction
- Disaster and development;
- Prevention and mitigation framework;
- Mainstreaming DRR in development planning;
- Disaster risk reduction practices.

Module 4: Disaster preparedness planning
- Overview of preparedness planning processes and concepts;
- Preparedness planning processes in key areas such as:
    - Setting up a preparedness planning committee;
    - Achieving agreement on preparedness arrangements;
    - Documenting preparedness arrangements;
    - Conducting preparedness training;
    - Testing preparedness arrangements.

Module 5: Emergency response
- Emergency response management principles and concepts;
- Key response implementation considerations;
- Use of emergency coordination centres;
- ICT in emergency responses.

Module 6: Disaster recovery
- Disaster recovery and reconstruction: concepts, practice and guidelines;
- Damage and loss estimation in recovery planning.

Module 7: Making disaster management work
- Cross-cutting considerations;
- Working with multi-agency teams;
- Policy, legal and institutional frameworks;
- Public communication;
- Media in disaster management.

Infectious disease disaster preparedness is another area in which well-coordinated capacity building efforts are required. Although the threat of pandemic H1N1 and H1N5 influenza were less severe than expected, the capacity building efforts to avert flu pandemic were impressive. The 266-page New York City's pandemic influenza preparedness and response plan has four aims: (a) limit severe illness and death from influenza; (b) work with health care partners to support appropriate influenza evaluations and care; (c) maintain essential medical services; (d) communicate rapidly, accurately and frequently with the public, the medical community and other stakeholders, using appropriate media. The nine capacity building areas in this document are: (1) command, control and management procedures; (2) surveillance and epidemiologic response; (3) laboratory diagnostics; (4) community control and response; (5) health care planning and emergency response; (6) delivery of antiviral drugs; (7) vaccine management; (8) mental health response; (9) communications. Each of these areas is rigorously addressed through adequate resourcing, infrastructure and workforce training.[15]

Capacity building for addressing terrorism-related disasters has attracted major international concern since the 11 September 2001 terror attacks. Due to the international dimension of terrorism the United States funds capacity building activities for nations like Pakistan which are likely to be havens for terror networks. Such capacity building efforts include military training, surveillance, emergency response and, increasingly, democratic reforms. America provided funding to the tune of $1 billion annually to Pakistan to fight terrorism between 2002 and 2008. Unfortunately, a major part of this capacity building money was diverted to fighting India in Kashmir, leaving thousands of Pakistani soldiers more vulnerable to Al Qaeda attacks. Internationally, much of the impetus driving capacity building assistance for counter-terrorism stems from the UN Security Council Counter-Terrorism Committee (CTC), which plays a central role in ensuring that states implement UN Security Council Resolution (UNSCR) 1373. The UN CTC determines the scope of what constitutes counter-terrorism capacity building assistance. The CTC also promotes coordination between international organisations engaged in providing this assistance or determining country needs. Seven important capacity building areas in relation to terrorism are: border security; transportation security; legislative, regulatory and legal policy development; legislative drafting, human rights and counter-terrorism training; law enforcement, security, military and intelligence training; chemical/biological/radiological/nuclear and explosives (CBRNE) terrorism prevention, mitigation, preparedness, response and recovery; Combating the financing of terrorism; cyber security and critical infrastructure protection.

The United Nations Global Counter-Terrorism Strategy was adopted by member states on 8 September 2006. The strategy, in the form of a resolution and an annexed Plan of Action (A/RES/60/288), is a unique global instrument that will enhance national, regional and international efforts to counter terrorism. This is the first time that all member states have agreed to a common strategic approach to fight terrorism, not only sending a clear message that terrorism is unacceptable in all its forms and manifestations but also resolving to take practical steps individually and collectively to prevent and combat it. The Resolution's Plan of Action entails: measures to address the conditions conducive to the spread of terrorism; measures to prevent and combat terrorism; measures to build states' capacity to prevent and combat terrorism and to strengthen the role of the United Nations system in this regard; measures to ensure respect for human rights for all and the rule of law as the fundamental basis of the fight against terrorism.[16]

Apart from being a cause of disasters, infectious diseases constitute a major risk following natural disasters. A comprehensive capacity building checklist for prevention and control of infectious diseases is provided by Kouadio *et al.* (Table 15.2).

Capacity building for these important areas of post-disaster infectious disease control need to be undertaken in an integrated and coordinated manner within a well-functioning health system, to maximise benefits. The situation in Haiti following the 2010 earthquake illustrates the limitations of vertical approaches to averting infectious diseases following disasters. Despite substantial donations of money and a large presence of volunteers and aid agencies, Haiti recorded its first outbreak of cholera in nearly a century, due, in part, to poor coordination of resources and a malfunctioning health system. As at December 2011, at least 5,000 Haitians have died and 300,000 became sick as a result of the infection. Addressing cholera in Haiti requires addressing the following areas: identify and treat all those with symptomatic cholera; make oral cholera vaccines available in Haiti and elsewhere; shore up Haiti's water system and improve sanitation; integrate cholera-specific projects into existing efforts to strengthen Haiti's health system; harmonise global health policy; and raise the bar on goals.[18]

Systems capacity building for emergency response should strive to achieve the 12 benchmarks, developed at the 2005 WHO regional meeting in Bangkok on Health Aspects of Emergency Preparedness and Response. These benchmarks included development of a legal framework in health emergency preparedness, regular updates of disaster management plans, rules of engagement for NGOs and other stakeholders in the event of an emergency, community mitigation processes, local capacity for emergency provision of essential services, capacity to identify risks and vulnerabilities at all levels, and maintenance of adequate human response capacity.[19]

So far, there has been significant progress with early detection systems in the Asia-Pacific region, but problems persist with dedicated emergency response staff and funding. As communities which are affected by emergencies tend to be cut off from the rest of the world, capacity building initiatives should focus also on improving community emergency preparedness, adaptation and resilience, particularly in high risk areas of flooding-prone nations like Bangladesh, Pakistan and the Philippines.

Table 15.2 Capacity building areas for infectious disease control following natural disasters

Prevention and control of infectious disease following natural disasters	Water-borne diseases			Air-borne/droplet diseases				Vector-borne diseases		Contamination from injury/wound	
	Diarrhoea (cholera; dysentery; others)	Leptospirosis	Hepatitis	ARI/ pneumonia/ influenza	Measles	Meningococcal meningitis	Tuberculosis	Malaria	Dengue fever	Tetanus	Cutaneous mucormycosis
Site planning	✓	–	–	✓	✓	✓	–	–	–	–	–
Clean water	✓	–	–	–	–	–	–	–	–	–	–
Good sanitation (e.g. excreta disposal)	✓	–	✓	–	–	–	–	–	–	–	–
Solid waste management	–	–	–	–	–	–	–	✓	✓	–	–
Water and food hygiene	✓	–	✓	–	–	–	–	–	–	–	–
Nutrition and supplements	–	–	–	–	✓	–	✓	–	–	–	–
Vaccination	–	–	–	–	✓	–	–	–	–	–	–
Vector control	–	–	–	–	–	–	–	✓	✓	–	–
Personal hygiene (e.g. hand washing)	✓	✓	✓	✓	–	–	✓	–	–	–	–
Personal protection	–	–	–	✓	–	–	–	✓	✓	–	–
Insecticide treated nets	–	–	–	–	–	–	–	✓	–	–	–
Isolation of the sick	–	–	–	✓	–	–	✓	–	–	–	–
Prophylactic treatment	–	–	–	–	–	–	–	✓	–	–	–
Wound/injury care	–	✓	✓	–	–	–	–	–	–	✓	✓
Health education	✓	✓	✓	✓	✓	✓	–	✓	✓	✓	✓
Disease management treatment and/or supportive care (follow national guidelines)	✓	–	–	✓	✓	✓	✓	✓	✓	✓	✓

Source: adapted from reference 17.

References

1 Shah, H. *Hurricane Katrina: Profile of a Super Cat.* New York: Risk Management Solutions, 2005.

2 Synolakis, C.E., Bernard, E.N. Tsunami science before and beyond Boxing Day 2004. *Philosophical Transactions of the Royal Society A,* 2006; 364: 2231–2265.

3 Rahu, M. Health effects of the Chernobyl accident: fears, rumours and the truth. *British Journal of Cancer,* 2003; 39: 295–299.

4 Pakistan Institute for Peace Studies. *Violence and Terrorism Report, 2010.* Islamabad: Pakistan, 2010.

5 Feeney, J.M., Wallack, M.K. Taking the terror out of terrorism. *Lancet,* 2011; 378: 851–852.

6 International Crisis Group. Sri Lanka: women's insecurity in the north and east. Asia Report Number 217, ICG, Brussels, 2011.

7 Haggard, S., Noland, M. Famine in North Korea Redux? *Journal of Asian Economics,* 2009; 20: 384–395.

8 United Nations Office for the Coordination of Humanitarian Affairs. Horn of Africa drought factsheet, 2011. Available from: http://reliefweb.int/sites/reliefweb.int/files/resources/Full_report_216.pdf (accessed 6 January 2011).

9 Chin, C., Sorenson, J., Harris, J.B. The origin of the Haitian cholera outbreak strain. *New England Journal of Medicine,* 2011; 364: 33–42.

10 Lloy, P.J., Weisel, C.P., Mellette, J.R. Characterisation of the dust/smoke aerosol that settled east of the World Trade Center (WTC) in Lower Manhattan after the collapse of the WTC 11 September 2001. *Environmental Health Perspectives,* 2002; 110: 703–714.

11 Inter-governmental Panel on Climate Change. Glossary Working Group, Annex 1, 2006.

12 International Committee of the Red Cross. *Climate Centre.* Geneva, ICRC, 2009.

13 Asian Disaster Preparedness Center. *Building Disaster Risk Reduction in Asia: A Way Forward.* Bangkok: ADPC, 2004.

14 Asian Disaster Preparedness Center. The 41st regional disaster management training course, Bangkok, Thailand, January to February 2012.

15 New York Department of Health and Mental Hygiene. *Pandemic Influenza Preparedness and Response Plan.* New York: NYDHMH, 2006.

16 United Nations General Assembly. Resolution 60/288: United Nations Global Counter-terrorism Strategy, New York, 2006.

17 Kouadio, I.K., Aljunid, S., Kamigaki, T., Hammad, K., Oshitani, H. Infectious diseases following natural disasters: prevention and control measures. *Expert Review of Anti-infective Therapy,* 2012: 10: 95–104.

18 Ivers, L.C., Farmer, P., Almazor, C.P., Leandre, F. Five complementary interventions to slow cholera: Haiti. *Lancet,* 2010; 376: 2048–2051.

19 World Health Organization. *Health-related Aspects of Emergency Preparedness and Response.* Bangkok: WHO, November 2005. Available from: www.searo.who.int/LinkFiles/Publication_&_Documents_Rep_HAEPR_Nov-05-SEA-EHA.pdf (accessed 1 April 2012).

16 Capacity building for efficient health care delivery to prisoners

Evolution of prisons

Incarceration in its various forms has been part of human penal systems since the development of warfare. Biblical records document conquering Roman armies led by General Titus who, in AD 70, killed thousands of Jews, imprisoned and subsequently sold hundreds of thousands of war prisoners into slavery in Egypt. Genghis Khan's Mongol empire incarcerated defeated opponents in dungeons during the thirteenth and fourteenth centuries. Slave plantations constituted virtual prisons, as were harems populated with captured women during the Ottoman era.[1,2] Contrary to a widely held belief that modern prisons evolved following the Protestant revolution and the rise of post-Renaissance nation states in the seventeenth century, Geltner's archival study of penal systems in fourteenth century Florence and Venice showed a much earlier and southern European origin.[3] He argued that many core features of the modern prisons – including administration, finance and the classification of inmates – were already developed by the end of the fourteenth century, and that incarceration as a formal punishment was far more widespread from this period onwards. It is plausible that Italian cities pioneered modern prison systems because of the Catholic Church's open advocacy for prisons to replace floggings and executions as punishment from the late thirteenth century onwards. By the mid-fifteenth century, prisons had become more widely used as a punishment option in Italian provinces, and were constructed as permanent government institutions in city centres, staffed with wardens and prison guards employed by the state. Italy's medieval prisons were divided into sections according to sex and social class, with new areas added later for the infirm and the insane. The social structures of the city-states were more or less retained within the prison walls.

Britain was another major player in the evolution of modern prisons. British prisons evolved in part due to advocacy by opinion leaders like Thomas More, who in his 1516 book entitled *Of the Best State of a Republic, and of the New Island Utopia* suggested an ideal socio-political system in which imprisonment serves as punishment, and an alternative to enslavement or death by execution. However, during that era, only private prisons – such as London's Newgate prison – which were run primarily as business concerns, existed. Ironically, prisoners were incarcerated in private prisons mainly for non-payment of debt, yet they had to pay for their lodging in these debtors' prisons. Following the passage of the Elizabethan Poor Law in 1601, Houses of Correction were established to punish the 'wandering poor', including beggars and vagrants, through forced labour. These workhouses eventually became de-facto prisons for petty criminals. From the late 1600s, transportation to British colonies provided alternatives to imprisonment of convicts. Broken old ships were used as floating prisons while convicts awaited transportation. Transportation to the United States ceased from the 1770s following America's War of Independence. Consequently Australia became the preferred destination for British convicts. Hulks and Houses of Correction served as prisons until the First Fleet, comprising nine ships, two naval vessels and 759 convicts, sailed from England to Port Jackson, Australia on 26 January 1788. Between 1788 and 1850 the English government transported over 162,000 convicts to Australia in 806 ships. In 1779 the first purpose-built British state prison, Millbank, was opened in London.[4]

In the United States, the focal points for prison evolution in the late eighteenth century were in Pennsylvania and New York. Under the leadership of William Penn, Pennsylvania's Quaker-inspired code abolished the death penalty for all crimes except murder, using instead imprisonment with labour and fines. In 1783, a group of prominent Pennsylvanian citizens, led by Benjamin Franklin and Benjamin Rush, organised a movement to reform the harsh penal code promulgated by British colonialists in 1718. The new penal laws they advocated substituted community labour service and imprisonment for previous severe punishments such as public floggings and executions. To accommodate prisoners, the Walnut Street Prison was built in Philadelphia in 1790, and it is considered the first American prison. However, reaction against the public display of convicts on the streets of the city and the disgraceful conditions in the Walnut Street jail led to the formation, in 1791, of the Philadelphia Society for Alleviating the Miseries of Public Prisons (a name it retained for 100 years, at which time it became the Pennsylvania Prison Society), the first of such societies in the world. In New York, Calvinists, led by Reverend Louis Dwight, bemoaned the state of New York's prisons, and by 1818 they had set motion the process that led to the establishment of Auburn prison. Like their Quaker counterparts in Pennsylvania, the Calvinists believed in inmate reformation through labour, reflection and solitary confinement, although they were more tolerant of harsh prison regimes than the Quakers. Completed in 1819, Auburn prison experimented with a variety of forms of solitary confinement. In 1822, the prison's agent established a discipline built on silent labour by day and solitary confinement by night.[5]

In France under the *Ancien Régime*, the control of undesirable behaviour was split up between the royal administration, the judicial apparatus and the family, along traditionally regulated lines. The most common punishment meted out during this era was *supplice* – torture. The end of torture as a form of punishment and the birth of modern penal systems in France were analysed by Michel Foucault in *Discipline and Punish*[6] as serving two purposes – sequestrating torture of the underclass – many of whom were imprisoned simply because they were long-term unemployed – from public view, and shifting the locus of punishment from the body to the soul. One of the first French prisons was the Bastille prison. Originating from the French word *Bastide*, meaning fortress, the Bastille was constructed in 1382 to defend the eastern wall of Paris from hostile forces. It was converted to a prison in 1725. When a revolutionary mob stormed the Bastille prison in 1789 and decapitated the prison's warden, De Launay, they aimed to tear down this potent symbol of feudal power. This brazen act of civil disobedience snowballed into the French Revolution, which led to further complex changes in the French penal system, from intensification of terror and torture of French citizens in and out of prison, to a progressively humane penal system from the late-1790s onwards.[7]

In Spain, with the emergence of the 'modern' Spanish Inquisition following a 1478 agreement between King Ferdinand of Aragon, Queen Isabella of Castile and Pope Sixtus IV, Inquisition prisons (*casa di penitencia*) were established to house those convicted of 'lesser' religious crimes. During this era, prisons were established as punishment to complement banishment, confiscation and death sentences that characterised the so-called ancient inquisition, which evolved since the time of Constantine the Great, the first Christian Roman emperor. Chief among the influences for development of the modern inquisition was hatred and envy of the Jews and Moors resident in Spain. Most were forced to convert to Christianity, and others were imprisoned on grounds of heresy.[8] Spanish prisons subsequently evolved along the same lines as Italian, British and French prisons.

The Mongols used imprisonment sparingly, perhaps because the Genghis Khan dynasty perceived imprisoned adversaries as potential threats. Genghis Khan was himself imprisoned for several years by rival ethnic rulers prior to his escape and re-emergence as leader of the Mongolian Empire. The Mongol emperors utilised imprisonment as punishment only for low risk criminals and political adversaries. Most individuals convicted under the Mongol penal system were executed or had their limbs amputated.[9]

In China, the first modern prison was established towards the end of the Qing Dynasty in Beijing in 1912. Named 'Beijing No. 1 prison', it was based on London's Pentonville prison architecture and operations. Prior to this era, punishment was by torture, death by execution, banishment and fines. As Chinese society evolved and the frequency of petty crimes committed by poor Chinese increased, the government sent envoys to

England to examine the British penal system in 1898. In setting up Pentonville-style prisons in China, they framed the 'silent system' as strongly overlapping with Confucian ethics of reformation, labour and repentance in confinement. In line with the 1908 Chinese penal code, imprisonment was one of the three options for punishment, the others being death and fines. The Cultural Revolution of Communist leader Mao Tse Tung stimulated the development of the Chinese Gulag – *Laogai* penal philosophy – which accorded high priority towards prisoner rehabilitation through institutionalised, forced, unpaid labour. Currently, China has one of the largest prison populations globally.[10]

The Russian empire's prison system was established around 1855 under the Tsar feudal rule. Ethnic Russians comprised only about 40 per cent of the huge Tsarist Empire. Mistrust and insecurity stimulated the construction of prisons to incapacitate suspected insurgents. The 1917 Lenin-led revolution facilitated a major expansion of the Russian prison system. Although Lenin referred to the Tsarist Russian empire as a 'prison of the peoples', the Soviet Gulag system proved to be more repressive than that developed by Lenin's predecessors. Tsars believed in their divine right of rule and consequently there was no freedom of choice for the people classified as 'outsiders'. Similarly, Russian communism was a repressive one-party 'democracy' which proved to be even more repressive under Stalin. The Gulag system was a network of forced labour camps that, at its peak, consisted of over 400 official prisons and held over two million inmates. First begun in 1919, the system really did not flourish until the 1930s when Stalin used it with extreme regularity as an instrument of state security and industrialisation policy. Transformed into virtual slave labourers, Russian prisoners under Stalin's rule completed huge architectural projects including, the White Sea–Baltic Canal, the Moscow–Volga Canal, the Baikal–Amur main railroad line, numerous hydroelectric stations, and hundreds of roads and industrial complexes. Prison conditions were extremely harsh. Prisoners received inadequate food rations and insufficient clothing, which made it extremely difficult to survive the bitterly cold winters, infectious diseases and long working hours. In the 1990s, under the leadership of Gorbachev, the camps' populations diminished substantially. In today's post-communist Russia, political prisoners have declined significantly in relation to total number of prisoners.[11]

Imprisonment was a relatively recent form of punishment in Muslim nations. During the Ottoman era, male 'enemies of the empire' were killed, enslaved or indoctrinated into military service (e.g. Janissary warriors from captured Christian territories). From the fifteenth century onwards, the established practice of killing all male relatives of a newly crowned Sultan in order to prevent succession rivalry was replaced by life imprisonment of potential rivals. Some historians posit that the policy of imprisonment contributed to the decline of the Ottoman Empire as opportunistic and politically inexperienced rivals of sitting sultans were rescued from prison by factional players and openly rebelled to facilitate their installation. The *Sharia* penal system was developed in part to reduce the need for imprisonment. To date, Muslim societies have among the lowest imprisonment rates in the world, with imprisonment a relatively modern but less popular addition to classic *Sharia* punishment options such as *diyeh* (fines and blood money, a popular penal sanction in Iran and Afghanistan).[12]

These diverse focal points of prison evolution served as templates for modern prisons globally. The British Empire introduced its penal system into most of its vast colonies. In Australia, the Port Arthur prison structure and function typify one such British colonial legacy (Figure 16.1).

Currently a tourist centre, the Port Arthur prison complex was established in 1833 to house British and Irish convicts who had re-offended in Australia. Its extensive 'separate' (or 'model') prison wing was designed in line with London's Pentonville prison. The separate system is a form of prison management based on the principle of solitary confinement, and enforced prohibition of communication when prisoners work in groups. When first introduced by the Eastern State Penitentiary, Philadelphia, in the early nineteenth century, the twin objective of such a prison or 'penitentiary' was that of reformation of prisoners through silent reflection, as well as enhanced prison security. The design of the separate wings of Pentonville and Port Arthur prisons was such as to minimise communication among prisoners. In most separate prison systems, prisoners were required to wear masks and were prohibited from communicating with one another even during communal exercise. Records indicate that a majority of prisoners developed severe mental illnesses and that a significant proportion

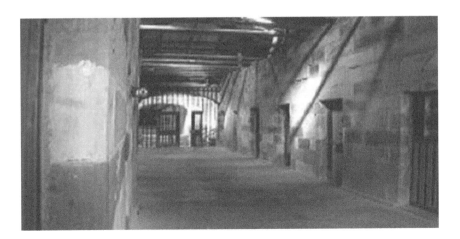

Figure 16.1 Separate prison section, Port Arthur, Tasmania (source: Wikipedia (common domain), available from: http://en.wikipedia.org/wiki/Port_Arthur,_Tasmania (accessed 2 April 2012)).

committed suicide as a result of austere prison conditions and lack of meaningful human contact.[13]

The British prison system was progressively introduced to India, Malaysia and other British colonies in Asia, Africa and the Middle East. The French, Spanish and Italian prison systems were also introduced to their vast colonies in Africa and South America. The Dutch introduced the British-style prison system into Indonesia and South Africa. In Indonesia's Batavia Retribution Museum, relics of the Dutch prison system, in the form of dungeons, are found, above which lived and worked prison officers.

The Russian prison structure was established in all colonies under the former Soviet Union, extending from Central Asia to Central Europe. The Chinese prison system developed as a blend of Confucian, British and Russian penal codes, and China currently runs the third most populated prison in the world. Prisons in contemporary Muslim nations evolved from a hybrid of *Sharia* and Western (colonial) influence, with imprisonment a less favoured penal option compared with punishments directed against the body.

John Howard, one of the pre-eminent prison health advocates of the eighteenth century, championed the introduction of prison health policies by carefully detailing the poor health conditions of British prisons and advocating for centralised action to better care for prisoners' health. His advocacy efforts facilitated the passage of the 1774 Health of Prisoners Act, which made statutory provisions for the health of the confined, the first such legislation for prisoners globally.[14]

As modern medicine developed, more health services were made available to prisoners. The provision of an expanded range of services created opposition among British opinion leaders who advocated a paternalistic

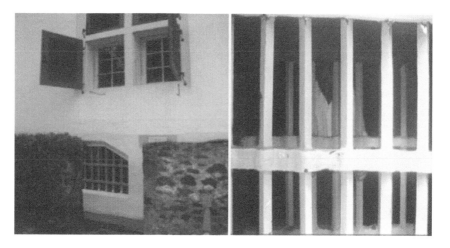

Figure 16.2 Batavia Retribution Museum, Jakarta, showing dungeon in the basement floor, and author in one of the dungeons, 2010.

and charity oriented approach to prison health policies. The public debate concerning how prisoners should be cared for created the setting for the first major prison policy in England – the Less Eligibility policy.

The main thrust of the Less Eligibility policy is that if imprisonment is to serve as a deterrent, the health and welfare care given to a prisoner should be of a lesser quality compared to that provided to a member of the lowest significant social class of a free society. This policy was adapted from the Less Eligibility Principle of English Poor Laws of the sixteenth century.[15] In many societies, this policy perspective is deeply ingrained in collective consciousness of civil society. The ideological right calls into effect the principle of Less Eligibility when it perceives inmates are enjoying the 'high life' in prison. The ideological left appeals to the prohibitions against cruel and unusual punishment, as well as the UN conventions on minimum standards for treatment of prisoners, when it perceives the penal regime to be too harsh.

The guiding principles of the Less Eligibility policy were propounded by Jeremy Bentham:

> If the condition of persons maintained without property by the labour of others were rendered more eligible than that of persons maintained by their own labour, then ... individuals destitute of property would be continually withdrawing themselves from the class of persons maintained by their own labour, to the class of persons maintained by the labour of others.[16]

This policy perspective was framed as a way of deterring crime by making health and welfare conditions in prison so bare as to discourage recidivism.

The Less Eligibility policy has been widely condemned by modern public health and prison policy experts as counterproductive and a threat to community health. For example, the 2003 Moscow Declaration on 'prison health as part of public health' advocates for prison health services to be of equivalent standard to those provided in the general community.[17] The Less Eligibility policy was implemented during an era when there was little understanding of the impact of social factors in causation of crime, and with little regard to the threat that unhealthy prisoners posed to the health of their immediate communities. Custodial authorities of the eighteenth century were primarily concerned with discouraging economic dependency of the underclass on the state. Using the Less Eligibility policy to address this concern is, at best, short-sighted. Nevertheless, this 'foundation policy' of prison health services continues to serve the objectives of penal populists who argue for more austere regimes in prison as a method of deterrence. It has hindered important reform measures related to prisoners' health promotion and rehabilitation, and needs to be continuously addressed if progressive prison reforms are to be sustainably implemented.

The evolution of prisons has important implications for the scope and quality of health services. The main manifest functions of prisons are punishment, retribution, incapacitation and rehabilitation. Health service provision and rehabilitation, in most prison settings, receive inadequate attention, especially when a potential conflict with security concerns exists. The policies implemented to address health care in prisons are influenced by myriad factors ranging from cost, nature of offenders, to the influence wielded by penal populists and relatives. In the United States, for example, the prisoner health care co-payment policy exemplifies an ideologically driven policy to reduce prisoner health care costs.

In 2000, the US Congress passed the Federal Prisoner Health Care Co-payment Act of 2000, with the stated primary purpose of 'combating over-utilisation of prison health care services and control rising prisoner healthcare costs'.[18] Congressman Matt Salmon summarised common arguments in favour of prisoner co-payments in a submission to the House Judiciary Crime Committee on 30 September 1999.[19] Below I list his arguments and my counter-arguments:

- Health care costs of federal prisoners in the US have risen from US$137.6 million in 1990 to US$354 million in 1998. Co-payment would exert downward pressure.

Counter-argument. Real prisoner health care cost increases are primarily a consequence of the rise in prison populations and not of increased per-prisoner provision. Between 1992 and 1998, the US imprisonment rate grew from 313 to 452 per 100,000 adult population, or to 680 per 100,000 if inmates in local jails are included.[20] In fact, although real national per capita health care costs have risen progressively from US$3,059 in 1990 to US$4,140 in 1999, real per capita federal inmates' health care costs were hardly any higher at the end of the period. They were US$3,001 in 1990, increased to a high of US$3,703 in 1996, and then decreased to US$3,242 by 1999.[21] Thus, there is already a downward pressure on per-prisoner health care costs, and hence relative levels of treatment. Co-payments may further reduce health care costs, but at the price of inferior health care services compared with that of the general community.

- By discouraging the overuse of health services through co-payment policy, prisoners in true need of attention will receive better care.

Counter-argument. Most prison surveys have shown that a majority of prisoners generally have a genuine need of enhanced health services.[22] A co-payment system might further widen health inequalities between poor prisoners and rich prisoners, and between prisoners and the general US population. A similar policy, Managed Health Care, which has been implemented in most southern and western state prisons in the US, has so far resulted in generally worse health care outcomes for 'inmates in true need of attention'.[23]

- Prisoner co-payment policies deter malingering inmates, thus reducing the stress of monitoring on (already overburdened) corrections officers.

Counter-argument. Those inmates who access prison health services out of boredom are unlikely to comply with prison regulations unless alternative outlets are provided. They may in fact create more stress for prison officers.

- The co-payment system may generate a modest income, which should cover the cost of its administration.

Counter-argument. A study by the California state auditor determined that the California Department of Corrections annual co-payment programme collection (US$5 per prisoner-initiated clinic visit) amounted to less than one-third (US$645,000) of the estimated annual collection (US$1.7 million) and that the estimated annual cost of administering the programme (US$3.2 million) amounted to almost five times the annual collection.[24]

- A co-payment policy does not deny inmates' constitutionally guaranteed access to health care. All co-payment systems have special provisions for free health care to those who do not have the means to pay.

Counter-argument. Studies have shown that the poor are highly sensitive to even minor health care co-payment costs.[25] In practice, health care co-payment policies position custodial authorities as intermediaries, thus impairing the actions and independence of prison health workers. This compromises the confidentiality of inmates' health status, with its potential repercussions.

It is noteworthy that, according to the United States Bureau of Justice Statistics' (BJS) 2010 prison report (http://bjs.ojp.usdoj.gov/content/pub/pdf/p10.pdf), for the first time since 1972, the US prison population had fallen from the previous year and that for the second year in a row the number of people under the supervision of adult correctional authorities had also declined. The overall US prison population at the end of 2010 was 1,605,127, a decrease of 9,228 prisoners or 0.6 per cent from year end 2009. The number of state prisoners declined by 0.8 per cent (10,881 prisoners). During 2010, prison releases (708,677) exceeded prison admissions (703,798) for the first time since BJS began collecting jurisdictional data in 1977.

Capacity building for improving prisoner health care

Sustainable capacity building for improving prisoner health care services requires the active participation of all major stakeholders – the international community, national governments, custodial authorities, prison health workers and prison inmates. Two such global initiatives are the UN minimum standards for the treatment of prisoners and the Moscow Declaration on prisoner health. The Standard Minimum Rules for the Treatment of Prisoners were adopted on 30 August 1955 by the United Nations Congress on the Prevention of Crime and the Treatment of Offenders, held at Geneva, and approved by the Economic and Social Council in resolutions of 31 July 1957 and 13 May 1977. Although not legally binding, the Standards provide guidelines for international and domestic law as regards persons held in prisons and other forms of custody. They set out what is generally accepted as being good principle and practice in the treatment of prisoners and the management of penal institutions. Section 12 of the Rules states: 'The sanitary installations shall be adequate to enable every prisoner to comply with the needs of nature when necessary and in a clean and decent manner.'[26] This Declaration is regularly relied on by prison advocacy groups, including the Red Cross Societies and Amnesty International in advocating on behalf of the incarcerated.

The Moscow Declaration on prison health as an integral part of public health was formulated at the 2003 Annual Meeting of the WHO European Network for Prisons and Health was held on 23–25 October 2003 in Moscow, Russia. During the meetings and conference, the delegates agreed to: (a) adopt a Declaration to draw attention to the importance of penitentiary health as an integral part of the public health system of any country; (b) establish a Task Force for Prisons and Health consisting of representatives of those organisations both national and non-governmental which have shown substantial and continuing activity in the area of prison health; (c) accept a Work Plan which included development of a scheme to recognise the work by staff in several prisons in Europe in promoting health in prisons and to encourage the use of those examples of good practice for the benefit of all countries; (d) to produce a Practical Guide to prison health.

The seminal prison health guide which resulted from the Moscow Declaration is entitled *Health in Prisons: WHO Guide to the Essentials of Prisoner Health.*[27] This important capacity building document proposes, in 14 chapters, programmes, policies and procedures for providing prisoners with optimal health care. It addresses infectious diseases like tuberculosis, mental health and managing stress among prison officers using approaches that may be adapted globally. Due in part to the advocacy efforts of the WHO (Europe) health in prisons project, capacity building for most of the initiatives proposed in this document have been implemented in most WHO Europe member states. Countries like the United Kingdom, Norway and France have integrated prison health care provision into their respective general health services.

Nationally, capacity building efforts need to reorient penal health care philosophy from Less Eligibility towards the 'equivalence' principle. Also, a better appreciation of basic social determinants of most prisoners' health will assist in development of appropriate policies and programmes.

National prison policies need to address priority problems of prisoners, not just those that may endanger the public such as HIV. For example, rape is a major hazard in most prison settings, which may result in major communicable and non-communicable disease consequences. A same-sex environment, sexually active age group, absence of strong social controls, impersonalisation of social relationships, prison culture, as well as the socio-demographic and personality traits of incarcerated individuals, tend to precipitate deviant sex conduct in prisons. Research into the subject of sex in prisons is fraught with major methodological, practical and ethical obstacles. Nevertheless, studies on this phenomenon, based on reports and meta-analysis from credible sources, may lead to better understanding of it and appropriate management. The potential health implications of non-consensual or illegal sexual contact in prison settings relate to both communicable diseases' transmission and psychiatric problems. Sexually transmissible diseases such as HIV infection and hepatitis B appear to be more efficiently transmitted via 'high risk' sexual acts such as unprotected anal sex, activities that are fairly common in male prison settings. In US prisons, the sexual activities most commonly associated with violence and infectious diseases risk are prison rape as well as sex between inmates and prison staff.

A book detailing numerous chilling instances of criminal sexual acts involving female inmates in US prisons was published by the Human Rights Women's Rights Project in 1996.[28] Most of the cases detailed in the book involved male prison officers and civilian staff engaged in sexual contacts with prisoners in women's prisons in California, Washington DC, Georgia, Illinois, Michigan and New York. The majority of female inmates were coerced into sexual activity using threats, or in exchange for contraband and favourable treatment. Although custodial authorities assert that sexual misconduct in prisons is viewed seriously, only a minority of accused staff were formally investigated during the review period.

Rape, defined as 'sexual acts between inmates that is accompanied by the use of threat of force or coercion, or the provision or denial of privileges among inmates'[29] is a recurring security and health issue in prison settings. It may occur in heterosexual or homosexual settings. In male homosexual rape, the sexual tension that may be precipitated by viewing naked co-prisoners in shower rooms, and the social meanings of roles adopted by masculine 'wolf' rapists, and their more feminine 'punk' victims in prison settings, may be influential. In some men's prisons, male rapists' aggressive, violent, sexual assaults are often excused on the grounds that rape is an expression of the perpetrators' manhood. In such prisons, victims are understandably reluctant to discuss attacks with custodial authorities and other inmates who tend to have more sympathy and understanding for the rapists, and who are often inclined to blame the victim for 'making himself vulnerable through his mannerisms'. Rape victims in such settings can rarely expect help in dealing with the feelings of degradation, fear, hatred and humiliation that result from the actual attack, or from discussions of it. Such situations precipitate psychological and mental health problems among victims.

The Prison Rape Elimination Act of 2003 was a major milestone in a centrally coordinated response to sexual violence in US prisons. It was promulgated in response to studies which indicate that there were 60,000–70,000 victims of prison sexual violence in US prisons every year over the past decade (Figure 16.3).

It is the first federal law to address sexual violence in prisons. Its provisions apply to all prisons, juvenile detention centres, jails and immigration detention centres in the United States. The Act states that sexual assault in detention can constitute a violation of the Eighth Amendment of the United States Constitution and requires that facilities adopt a zero-tolerance approach to this form of abuse. The law calls for the development of national standards about how to address prisoner rape, the gathering of nationwide statistics about the problem, the provision of grants to states to combat it and the creation of a review panel to hold

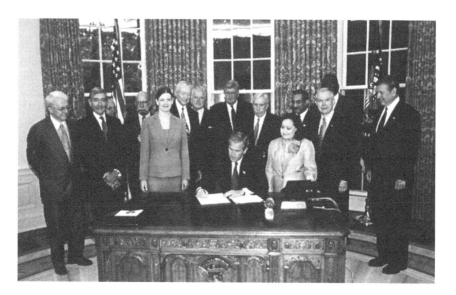

Figure 16.3 President Bush signing the unanimously passed Prison Rape Elimination Act into Law on 4 September 2003 (source: Reuters (public domain)).

annual public hearings with the best and the worst performing corrections facilities nationwide. The passage of the Prison Rape Elimination Act (PREA) was a vitally important advance in the effort to end sexual violence behind bars, and the first few years of PREA implementation have brought significant attention to this type of abuse.

In 2006, the Justice Policy Centre of the Urban Institute published a landmark report on innovative practices adopted by custodial authorities following the promulgation of the 2003 Rape Act, to address sexual violence in US prisons.[30] With regard to preventing sexual violence, the major highlights of the report were:

- Thirty-five states reported having policies and programmes to prevent sexual violence in prisons. The most frequently cited preventative measures included inmate housing assignment and transfer strategies, initiatives to address overcrowding and inmate education.
- A common theme that served as the foundation for many states' new policies and procedures regarding sexual violence is a commitment at the most senior levels of the department to change the correctional culture, thereby affecting the attitudes of staff and inmates.
- Some states put together security review teams, mapping systems and surveillance strategies to identify and address facility design vulnerabilities.
- All states have inmate classification systems for making housing decisions, and some use these systems to prevent sexual violence by identifying potential victims and perpetrators of sexual violence.
- Unit management procedures, such as special staffing approaches for dealing with problems that inmates may face, have been employed to prevent sexual violence.
- Many states have specific inmate education or awareness campaigns about sexual violence – how to prevent it, how to identify vulnerabilities and what to do if one becomes victimised.
- A small number of states use peer education and mentoring programmes to help prevent sexual violence.

In relation to investigation and prosecution:

- Thirty-eight states reported having policies and programmes in place to investigate reports of prison sexual violence and prosecute cases as appropriate.
- Across prisons, official policies or protocols include many similar elements, such as response to incidents that occurred in the past, immediate response to recent incidents, separation of the victim and perpetrator, securing the crime scene, evidence collection from perpetrators and victims, chain of command and notification requirements, and reporting and documentation requirements.

- States use different resources to implement the investigation process. In many states, investigation of allegations of prison sexual violence is the responsibility of wardens, other facility managers or investigators assigned to specific facilities. Other states use external agencies, such as the state highway patrol or the county law enforcement agency to investigate. States' policies regarding which agency leads the investigative process may vary depending on whether the perpetrator is an inmate or a department employee or volunteer.
- A number of states identified the importance of community medical facilities' involvement in administering rape kits to collect forensic evidence.

Prior to proclamation of the 2003 Rape Act, it was not clear the extent to which state departments of corrections were addressing sexual violence in systematic ways. In fact, little information existed about what strategies were being put into practice in prison systems across the country. Subsequently, mandatory recordkeeping and a push for eliminating sexual violence incidents in prisons has moved many custodial authorities to develop specific responses to prison sexual violence or to further refine approaches already in place. Consequently, the (reported) incidence of prison sexual violence has reduced significantly in US prisons.

The Prison Rape Elimination Act also legalised the creation of the National Prison Rape Elimination Commission, whose mandate was to study the problem more qualitatively and devise national standards for its detection, prevention and response. Doing so proved to be a slow process, as it was not until June 2009 that the Commission published its recommendations. The Commission set performance indicators for all prisons, jails, juvenile detention centres and immigration detention centres in relation to prison rape. One of the Commission's most important standards requires that all inmates be screened in order 'to assess their risk of being sexually abused by other inmates or sexually abusive toward other inmates'. The main concern expressed by opponents of the Commission's standards is that observing them will be too expensive. One Prison Rape Elimination Act provision barred the Commission and the Attorney General from establishing standards 'that would impose substantial additional costs compared to costs currently expended by Federal, State, and local prison authorities'. However, the broad-based support received by the Act has so far limited the impact of its opponents. If approved by the US government, state custodial authorities are not required to comply with the Commission's standards but those that do not risk a 5 per cent federal prison funding decrease.

The implementation of state-based policies to prevent prison sexual violence post-2004 has, so far, not eliminated incidents of sexual assault in US prisons. Indeed, the 2007 prison sexual assault report by the Justice Department – 'Sexual Victimization in State and Federal Prisons Reported by Inmates, 2007' – documented that 4.5 per cent of the state and federal prisoners surveyed reported sexual victimisation in the past 12 months. Given a national prison population of 1,570,861, the report suggests that, in 2007 alone, more than 70,000 prisoners were sexually abused. Prison rape is not inevitable, but it is all too predictable when prison authorities fail to develop adequate administrative and human resources capacity to enforce a zero-tolerance policy on sexual abuse.

What the US Rape Elimination Act seems to be achieving well so far is the establishment of an effective monitoring, evaluation and management framework to facilitate national comparisons of sexual assaults, categorise them and work in partnership with custodial authorities to stimulate strategies and programmes for improvement. For example, the 2007 Justice Department report indicated that five of the ten prison facilities with the highest reported rates of inmate-on-inmate victimisation are in Texas, with reported prevalence ranging from 3.3 to 8.8 per cent. Texas has a crowded state prison system with a long and notorious history of prison violence, marked by staff indifference to, and complicity with, abuse. Such comparisons were not easily available prior to the promulgation of the 2003 Rape Act. All inmates have the right be treated with dignity. No matter what crime someone has committed, sexual violence must never be part of a prison penalty.

Currently, however, the government is being pressured by custodial officers to weaken the standards suggested by the Commission, based on their assessment that the changes will cost too much to implement. If the Obama administration needlessly delays in approving these standards, or strips them of their force because of pressure from corrections leaders, then tens of thousands of men, women and children will continue to be raped while in the government's care, when such sexual violence could have been prevented.

Custodial authorities and prison health workers have a lot to contribute with regards to capacity building of prison health services. Controversy exists about the suitability of having prison health workers operate under the correctional banner or under the purview of respective health departments. The current consensus is that, in the interests of health professionals' autonomy as well as achievement of equivalence principle of health care provision, prison health services should be integrated with the general health services. The scope of health services should be expanded from the hitherto narrow model of medical care to a more comprehensive model of health care provision comprising allied health workers such as psychologists, social workers and epidemiologists. Integrated service linkage arrangements should be instituted such that inmates are able to access adequate health services in the community while in prison, and following release. The quality, quantity and distribution of prison health workers are sub-optimal in most nations. Standards for correctional staff in many nations are generally inferior to those in the general community. The quantity of health workers is also generally low, when compared to the co-morbid conditions common among prisoners. Due in part to economies of scale, it is rare for rural prisons to be adequately well staffed. Building capacity for national and local prison human resources and management entails development of national minimum standards, such as those developed for Australian prisons.[31]

Also important is the need to co-opt prisoners to contribute to the capacity building efforts through participation in decision making, as well as in research. Prisoners are uniquely positioned to provide vital 'bottom-up' information regarding the quality, quantity and distribution of prison health services. The use of robust research methods in accessing prisoners' perspectives is also important.[32]

Prisons constitute an important barometer of health equity in most societies. Correctional settings represent an opportunity to address health problems among those who may not be able to easily access or afford health services in the general community. Advocacy for capacity building for improved health services need to emphasise major positive public health benefits of addressing prisoner health services. Adequate funding is important, and advocacy for adequate correctional health care funding should be implemented concurrently with framing prisons as a last resort for criminal justice. Human resources gaps need to be addressed. The health care service for prisoners is a small, isolated service that is seen as an unattractive place to work. The work need not be unattractive – much is fascinating, based on the author's decade-long work experience as a public health officer in Australian prisons. Finally, appropriate prison architecture has a strong potential to contribute to prisoner health improvement efforts.[33]

References

1 Lane, G. *Ghengis Khan and Mongol Rule*. Westport, CT: Greenwood Publishing Group Inc., 2004.
2 Swanson, G.W. The Ottoman police. *Journal of Contemporary History*, 1992; 7: 243–260.
3 Geltner, G. *The Medieval Prison: A Social History*. Princeton, NJ: Princeton University Press, 2008.
4 Morris, N., Rothman, D.J. *The Oxford History of the Prison*. New York: Oxford University Press, 1995.
5 Graber, J. 'When friends had the management it was entirely different': Quakers and Calvinists in the making of New York prison discipline. *Quaker History*, 2008; 97: 19–40.
6 Foucault, M. *Discipline and Punish: The Birth of the Prison*. New York: Knopf Doubleday Publishing Company, 1989.
7 Chantraine, G. French prisons of yesteryear and today: two conflicting modernities – a socio-historical view. *Punishment and Society*, 2010; 12: 27–47.
8 Griffiths, A., Griffiths, M.A. *Spanish Prisons*. New York: Bibliobazaar, 2009.
9 Lane, G. *Daily Life in the Mongol Empire*. New York: Greenwood Publishing Inc., 2006.
10 Wu, M.H. *Laogai: The Chinese Gulag*. New York: Westview Press, 1992.
11 Applebaum, A. *Gulag: A History of the Soviet Camps*. London: Penguin Press, 2003.

12 Shaw, E.J., Shaw, S.K. *History of Ottoman Empire and Modern Turkey: Volume 2, Reform, Revolution, and Republic: The Rise of Modern Turkey 1808–1975.* Cambridge: Cambridge University Press, 1997.

13 Weidenhiofer, M. *Port Arthur: A Place of Misery.* London: Oxford University Press, 1981.

14 MacDonald, J.M. John Howard; prison reformer. *American Journal of Psychiatry,* 1959; 115: 852–853.

15 Sieh, E.W. Less eligibility: the upper limit of penal policy. *Criminal Justice Policy Review,* 1989: 3: 159–183.

16 Bentham, J. *Bentham Papers: Copies of Essays of 1796.* London: British Museum, 1796.

17 World Health Organization. *Moscow Declaration: Prison Health as part of Public Health.* Moscow: WHO, 24 October 2003.

18 Federal Prisoner Health Care Co-payment Act of 2000, Pub. L. No. 106–294, 12 October 2000. United States 106th Congress.

19 Federal Prisoner Health Care Co-payment Act. Representative Matt Salmon, House Subcommittee, 30 September 1999. Washington, DC: US House of Representatives, Committee on the Judiciary.

20 Zimring, F.E., Kamin, S., Hawkins, G. *Crime and Punishment in California: The Impact of Three Strikes and You're Out.* Berkeley, CA: Institute of Governmental Studies, University of California, 1999, pp. 1–12.

21 United States General Accounting Office (GAO). Containing the health care costs for an increasing inmate population. Testimony by Richard Stana before the United States Senate Subcommittee on Criminal Justice Oversight. Washington, DC: GAO, 6 April 2000.

22 National Commission on Correctional Health Care (NCCHC). *The Health Status of Soon-to-be-released Inmates: A Report to Congress.* Chicago, IL: NCCHC, 2002.

23 Robbins, I.P. Managed health care in prison as cruel and unusual punishment. *Journal of Law and Criminology,* 1999; 99: 195–238.

24 Birdlebough, S. Analysis of SB 396: health care for prisoners, Sacramento, letter in support of SB 396, on behalf of Friends Committee on Legislation in California, 11 July 2001.

25 The 50 Years is Enough Network (T50YEN). Empty promises: the IMF, World Bank, and the planned failures of global capitalism. Washington, DC: T50YEN, Jurist 1 July 2005.

26 United Nations, Standard minimum rules for the treatment of prisoners, 30 August 1955. Available from: www.unhcr.org/refworld/docid/3ae6b36e8.html (accessed 7 January 2012).

27 World Health Organization. *Health in Prisons: WHO Guide to the Essentials of Prisoner Health.* Copenhagen: WHO Europe, 2007.

28 Human Rights Watch. All too familiar-sexual abuse of women in U.S. state prisons, Human Rights Watch, New York, 1996.

29 Awofeso, N. Sex in prisons: a management guide. *Australian Health Review,* 2002; 25: 149–158.

30 Zweig, J.M., Naser, R.L., Blackmore, J., Schaffer, M. *Addressing Sexual Violence in Prisons: A National Snapshot of Approaches and Highlights of Innovative Strategies.* Washington, DC: Urban Institute, 2006.

31 Belcher, J., Yaman, F.A. *Prisoner Health in Australia: Contemporary Information Collection and a Way Forward.* Canberra: AIHW, 2007.

32 Reed, J., Lyne, M. The quality of health care in prison: results of a year's programme of semi-structured inspections. *British Medical Journal,* 1997; 315: 1420–1424.

33 Awofeso, N. Unlocked potential: improving inmates' health through prison architecture. *International Journal of Prisoner Health,* 2011; 7: 3–9.

17 Capacity building for improved occupational health and safety

Evolution of occupational health and safety services

The International Labour Organization (ILO) defined occupational diseases as having a specific or a strong relation to occupation generally with only one causal agent. The main elements present in the definition of an occupational disease are: (a) the causal relationship between exposure in a specific working environment or work activity and a specific disease and (b) the fact that the disease occurs among a group of exposed workers with a frequency higher than that observed in other workers or in the general population.[1] This definition is distinguished from that of work-related diseases – with multiple causal agents, where factors in the work environment may play a role, together with other risk factors, in the development of such diseases, which have a complex aetiology. Diseases affecting working populations, defined as without causal relationship with work, such as back pain, but which may be aggravated by occupational hazards to health are further distinguished from occupational diseases.[2] Currently, 1.9–2.3 million deaths annually are attributed to occupation, 1.6 million deaths attributed to work-related diseases and 217 million cases of occupational diseases are documented globally every year.[3]

Mining evolved as one of humanity's oldest industries as hunter-gatherers sought appropriate stones and minerals to hunt, farm and fight. Most of the miners of the earlier eras were captured slaves. Occupational safety was not considered part of the occupation. From the beginning of the industrial revolution in Europe, mining gradually became a skilled occupation, attracting free citizens and artisans. In the sixteenth century, Paracelcius (1493–1541), a German-Swiss physician, authored a seminal document entitled *On the Miners' Sickness and Other Diseases of Miners*, which documented the occupational hazards of metalworking including treatment and prevention strategies. He was the first to determine that lead, arsenic and carbon monoxide, inhaled or ingested in high enough doses, may poison and kill miners. Bernardino Ramazzini (1633–1714), occupational and industrial health research pioneer, published in 1700, his most famous book, *De Morbis Artificum Diatriba* (Diseases of Workers), which represents the first comprehensive publication to address occupational diseases. In Chapter 14, entitled 'Diseases of Cleaners of Privies and Cesspits', Ramazzini posited that what is today known as hydrogen sulphide is responsible for odour, respiratory problems, corrosion of copper pipes and eye irritation in sewerage plants.

Industrial Britain laid the foundation for modern occupational health and safety. The repeal of a ban making trade unions illegal in 1824 stimulated workers' grassroots activism, and increased advocacy for occupational health and safety. Most factories in Manchester during the 1800s were unsanitary. Workers usually slept in their factories. The typhus outbreak in the cotton mills at Radcliffe Bridge of 1784 drew Manchester physician Thomas Pervical's attention to the sordid conditions of the factories and he initiated industrial legislation. In 1883, the first workers compensation act in Europe was passed by a Bismarck (Germany) parliament. By 1898, Thomas Legge was appointed the first Medical Inspector of Factories, thus facilitating the provision of statutory medical service for factory workers.

Percivali Pott (1714–1788) published the first known case of occupational cancer, among young chimney sweeps in the Britain. An act of Parliament was passed in 1840 to provide that after 1 July 1842, no sweep under the age of 21 years should climb a chimney. From 1911 to 1935, out of a population of 5,274 chimney sweepers there were 100 deaths from cancer of the scrotum, a much higher incidence than in other occupations. By 1852, alternative methods of heating, improved hygiene in the trade of chimney sweepers and improved methods of cleaning chimneys led to the near-total eradication of this cancer, now known to be caused by tar: 3,4-benzopyrene. This finding stimulated research in occupational diseases, for prevention, risk reduction and compensation purposes. Six industrial diseases were listed in the first compilation of this category of diseases in 1913. The ILO was created in 1919. Its first major activity was to declare anthrax an occupational disease. The list of diseases increasingly widened as societal work patterns became more sophisticated. The United Kingdom's 1974 Occupational Health and Safety Act was a major advance in prioritising prevention of occupational diseases, prompt management and rehabilitation/compensation. The World Health Organization Expert Committee on Identification and Control of Work-related Diseases met in Geneva from 28 November to 2 December 1983 and developed the concept of 'Occupational Health Programmes', aimed to protect and promote the health of workers. The document highlighted that 5–10 per cent of workers have some form of occupational health problems.[4] The *Whitehall 2* study also made important contributions to the evolution of occupational health and safety.[5] The final sample of non-industrial workers was 6,900 men and 3,414 women aged 35–55 in the London offices of 20 civil service departments, studied since 1985. The study showed that workers in the highest occupational categories had lower rates of hypertension and ischaemic heart disease, and a fourfold lower risk of mortality from such conditions compared with workers in the lowest industrial categories (Figure 17.1).

In 2003, the ILO published a global strategy on occupational health and safety. Section 15 of this document is particularly pertinent to this chapter, as it focusses on how ILO may assist nations in developing adequate capacity for disaster preparedness.[6]

A prime objective of capacity building for occupational health and safety is to develop healthy workplaces, defined as:

> one in which workers and managers collaborate to use a continual improvement process to protect and promote the health, safety and well-being of all workers and the sustainability of the workplace by considering the following, based on identified needs:
>
> - health and safety concerns in the physical work environment;
> - health, safety and well-being concerns in the psychosocial work environment, including organization of work and workplace culture;
> - personal health resources in the workplace and ways of improving the health of workers, their families and other members of the community.[7]

The business case for health workplaces is quite straightforward (Figure 17.2).

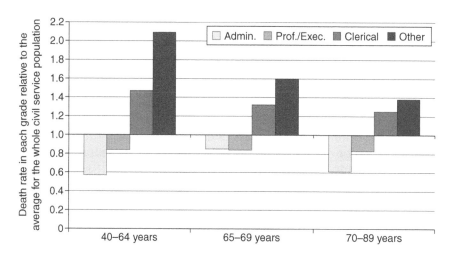

Figure 17.1 Death rate and employment grade over a 25-year period in men – Whitehall studies (adapted from reference 5).

Note
Average for the whole civil service population is set at 1.

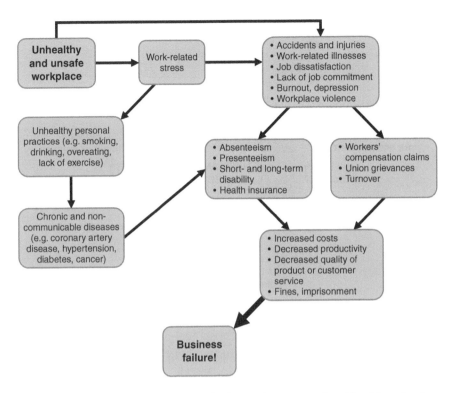

Figure 17.2 Summary of business case for improving occupational health and safety (adapted from reference 6).

Currently, nations which have developed adequate capacity to address occupational health and safety problems, such as Australia, have lower occupational diseases compared with nations like China and other developing nations where such capacities are weak. In developing nations, perverse incentives and moral hazard have contributed to increases in occupational claims by staff who wish to take advantage of generous compensation packages for occupational diseases, a situation being addressed by stiff fines to employees who fail to put in place adequate prevention and training measures.

Healthy workplaces: key action areas

Physical work environment

Occupational health and safety (OHS) issues in this domain include: chemical hazards (e.g. tobacco smoke), physical hazards (e.g. noise), biological hazards (e.g. malaria), ergonomic hazards (e.g. heavy lifting),

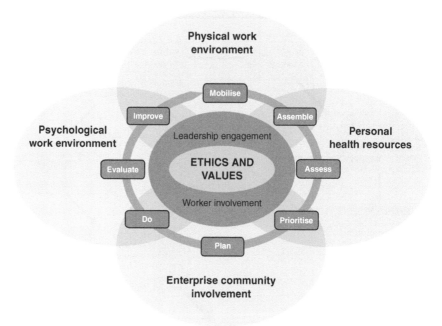

Figure 17.3 Key action areas for facilitating healthy workplaces (adapted from reference 6).

sanitary hazards (e.g. poor water and hygiene quality), mechanical hazards (machine hazards related to cranes), climatic hazards (e.g. excessive sun exposure), energy hazards (e.g. electric shock), transport hazards (e.g. driving on ice or poorly maintained vehicles).

Psychosocial work environment

OHS issues include poor work organisation (problems with work demands, time pressure, decision latitude, reward and recognition, support from supervisors, job clarity, job design, poor communication), lack of support for work–life balance, fear of job loss related to mergers, acquisitions, reorganisations or the labour market economy. In this regard, the Job Strain Model posits that increases in the risk of psychological and physical illness increases when work demands exceed the workers' job control (i.e. decision making capacity) and social/technical support from supervisors and colleagues.[8]

Personal health resources

Stress management is an important personal health resource to minimise the risk of work-related disorders such as depression, anxiety and burnout.

Studies show that employees with high levels of work-related stress experience higher levels of absenteeism and have higher levels of mental illness.[9] Work organisation issues which may tax personal health resources include: physical inactivity may result from long work hours, cost of fitness facilities or equipment, and lack of flexibility in when and how work breaks can be taken; poor diet may result from lack of access to healthy snacks or meals at work, lack of time to take breaks for meals, lack of refrigeration to store healthy foods or lack of knowledge; smoking may be allowed or enabled by workplace environments, particularly in developing nations.

Social responsibility

Social responsibility is an ethical obligation for organisations to benefit not only their stakeholders, but also the society at large. From an OHS perspective, extra-remuneration benefits to stakeholders might include extending free or subsidised primary health care to workers and their families, and subsidising public transportation and bicycles for employees to ride to work. At the community level, sponsorship of community events such as Health and Safety Week, and initiating activities to control pollution emissions and safely dispose of health hazards from work activities, are important aspects of social responsibility. Increasingly, public health acts and health impact assessments are being used to legislate and structure social responsibility activities of organisations.[10]

Building capacity to improve occupational health and safety

The first step in capacity building in occupational health and safety is to determine its scope – sun exposure, noise, biochemical hazards, airborne hazards, biological materials, dermal hazards, psychological hazards – and the extent to which major aspects apply to specific organisations as well as the adequacy of control measures.[11]

With regards to airborne hazards in the workplace, for example, a self-reported study of 4,500 Australian workers in a dozen major occupations revealed that 42 per cent of all participants believed they were exposed to airborne hazards (Figure 17.4). In about 22 per cent of organisations surveyed, nothing was done to address the self-reported workplace airborne hazard at the time of the survey.

Successful capacity building to address OHS hazards relies heavily on the adequacy and enforcement of workplace OHS laws. In nations like Australia where such laws are strictly applied and employers are fined for perceived negligence,[12] major OHS incidents have shown a downward decline. In contrast, nations like China which ineffectively operate weak OHS laws have generally recorded worsening workplace injury and fatality rates. At the organisational level, capacity building for creating healthy workplaces and reducing OHS hazards may be addressed from four perspectives:

- *Engineering controls*: e.g. eliminating hazards such as toxins, better machines, enclosing adverse work operations, improved ventilation, environmental monitoring of air quality and noise.
- *Safer work practices*: e.g. use of staff education and training as well as organisational OHS policies to improve work safety and occupational architecture, inspection and maintenance of processes, facilities and equipment used in organisations, prohibiting eating, drinking, smoking in regulated areas, employee-centred supervision and house-keeping services.
- *Administrative controls*: e.g. development of OHS committees to provide a framework for continuous safety improvements, limit exposure time to hazards e.g. worker rotations, scheduling operations with fewest employees needed, prevent fatigue, apply practical ergonomics principles, adequate supply of safety signs and equipment, accessibility to effective and well maintained personal protective equipment in relation to potential hazards, effective workplace emergency response plans.

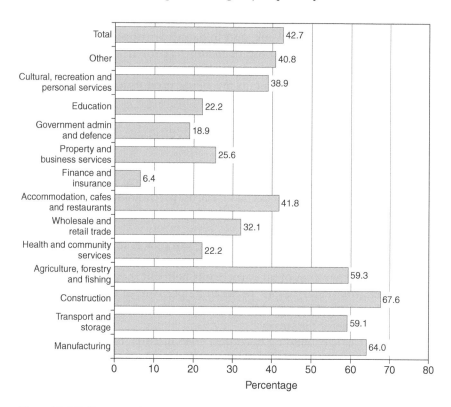

Figure 17.4 Self-reported exposure to airborne hazards in Australia workplaces (adapted from reference 10)

Note
N = 4,500.

- *Legislative controls*: where feasible, promulgate laws to enforce OHS strategies. The most common enforcement mechanism is through occupational health and safety acts. For example, the New South Wales Smoke-free Environment Act 2000 prohibits smoking in workplaces, and legalises sanctions, including fines for employers who contravene provisions of the Act. At the University of Western Australia, the Governing Council approved a law making all campuses of the university smoke free. In Australia, all states have compulsory workplace health and safety laws (e.g. OHS Act and Environment Act), and fines apply to organisations that contravene such Acts.

References

1 International Labour Organization. *Identification and Recognition of Occupational Diseases: Criteria for Incorporating Diseases into the ILO List of Occupational Diseases.* Geneva: ILO, 2009.
2 International Labour Organization. *Glossary of Definitions.* Geneva: ILO, 1993.
3 Holness, L. *Historic Perspective on Occupational Disease.* Toronto: Centre for Research Expertise in Occupational Disease, 2008.
4 World Health Organization. *Identification and Control of Work-Related Diseases: Report of Expert Committee.* Geneva: WHO, 1986.
5 Ferrie, J.E. (ed.). *Work Stress and Health: The Whitehall 2 Studies.* London: Cabinet office, 2004.
6 International Labour Organization. *Global Strategy on Occupational Health and Safety.* Geneva: ILO, 2003.
7 Burton, J. *World Health Organization Healthy Workplace Framework and Model.* Geneva: WHO, 2010.
8 Noblet, A. Building health promoting work settings: identifying the relationships between work characteristics and occupational stress in Australia. *Health Promotion International*, 2003; 18: 351–359.
9 Stansfeld, S., Candy, B. Psychosocial work environment and mental health: a meta-analytic review. *Scandinavian Journal of Work Environment and Health*, 2006; 32: 443–462.
10 Mittlemark, MB. Promoting social responsibility for health: health impact assessment and healthy public policy at the community level. *Health Promotion International*, 2001; 16: 269–274.
11 Miller, P., Kong, C. *Occupational Disease Exposures in Australia: Workers tell their Own Story.* Canberra: Comcare Conference, 2008.
12 Government of New South Wales. Occupational Health and Safety Act 2000 No. 40. Sydney: NSW, 2000.

18 Capacity building for improving mental health service delivery

Mental illness: scope and risk factors

Definitions of mental illness are notoriously difficult to draft. If they are framed too narrowly they deny services to people. If they are too broad they may result in unnecessary intervention. The ICD-10 definition – 'a general term which implies the existence of a clinically stigmatising set of symptoms associated with distress ... and with ... interference with personal functions' – and classification of diseases that fall under the rubric of mental illness exemplify a broad definitional approach, while the New South Wales 1990 Mental Health Act definition (Schedule 1) is narrow, as it excludes less severe, but common, forms of mental illness such as anxiety disorders:

> mental illness is defined as a condition characterised by the presence of symptoms such as delusions, hallucinations, serious disorder of thought form, a severe disturbance of mood, or sustained or repeated irrational actions, which seriously impairs, either temporarily or permanently, the mental functioning of a person

The American Medical Association's 2000 DSM-IV description of mental illness appears to strike the right balance:

> A clinically significant behavioral or psychological syndrome or pattern that occurs in an individual and that is associated with present distress ... or disability ... or with a significantly increased risk of suffering death, pain, disability, or an important loss of freedom.

The history of mental illness management dates back to 5000 BC, as evidenced by trephined skulls. Early humans widely believed that mental illness was the result of supernatural phenomena such as spiritual or demonic possession, sorcery, the evil eye or an angry deity and so responded with equally mystical, and sometimes brutal, treatments, including crude brain surgery. From the mid-seventeenth century presumed mentally ill people were imprisoned in asylums as punishment for, and to reverse, their choice of 'unreason'. Philippe Pinel (1745–1826) introduced 'moral care' for mentally ill Parisians. His new concepts of the care of the mentally ill were published in Pinel's *Traité medico-philosophique sur l'aliénation mentale* (1801; *Treatise on Insanity*, 1806). French physicians Thuillier and Deniker discovered Chlorpromazine, the first effective antipsychotic, introduced in 1952. However, improvements in the care for the mentally ill have not developed uniformly in all regions of the world, and most developing nations are still in the 'dark ages' of using alleged sorcery cures and chaining mentally ill as major treatment approaches.[1]

Major classes of mental illness as per the ICD-10 definition are:

F0   Organic, including symptomatic, mental disorders
F1   Mental and behavioural disorders due to use of psychoactive substances
F2   Schizophrenia, schizotypal and delusional disorders
F3   Mood [affective] disorders
F4   Neurotic, stress-related and somatoform disorders
F5   Behavioural syndromes associated with physiological disturbances and physical factors
F6   Disorders of personality in adult persons
F7   Mental retardation
F8   Disorders of psychological development
F9   Behavioural and emotional disorders with onset usually occurring in childhood and adolescence
F10 Unspecified mental disorders.

According to a 2010 World Health Organization report, by 2009, neuro-psychiatric disorders such as schizophrenia, depression, epilepsy, dementia, alcohol dependence and other mental, neurological and substance-use (MNS) disorders accounted for 13 per cent of the Global Burden of Disease, second only to infectious disorders (23 per cent), and are bigger burden than AIDS, TB and malaria combined (10 per cent). Mental illness burden currently surpasses both cardiovascular disease and cancer (Table 18.1).

Risk factors for mental illness vary widely depending on the mental health condition. For example, risk factors for schizophrenia – a devastating psychiatric syndrome with a median lifetime prevalence of 4.0 per 1,000 and a morbid risk of 7.2 per 1,000 – include: genetics,[3] age – young adults; gender – males; social adversity and prenatal malnutrition. A recent follow-up study following hospitalisation for cannabis-related illness revealed that cannabis use is associated with an adverse course of psychotic symptoms in schizophrenia, and vice versa, even after taking into account other clinical, substance use and demographic variables.[4]

Table 18.1 Burden of diseases due to mental illness-related conditions

Rank	Worldwide		High income countries[1]		Low and middle income countries	
	Cause	DALYs[2] (millions)	Cause	DALYs (millions)	Cause	DALYs (millions)
1	Unipolar depressive disorders	65.5	Unipolar depressive disorders	10.0	Unipolar depressive disorders	55.5
2	Alcohol-use disorder	23.7	Alzheimer's and other dementias	4.4	Alcohol-use disorder	19.5
3	Schizophrenia	16.8	Alcohol-use disorder	4.2	Schizophrenia	15.2
4	Bipolar affective disorder	14.4	Drug-use disorders	1.9	Bipolar affective disorder	12.9
5	Alzheimer's and other dementias	11.2	Schizophrenia	1.6	Epilepsy	7.3
6	Drug-use disorders	8.4	Bipolar affective disorder	1.5	Alzheimer's and other dementias	6.8
7	Epilepsy	7.9	Migraine	1.4	Drug-use disorders	6.5
8	Migraine	7.8	Panic disorder	0.8	Migraine	6.3
9	Panic disorder	7.0	Insomnia (primary)	0.8	Panic disorder	6.2
10	Obsessive-compulsive disorder	5.1	Parkinson's disease	0.7	Obsessive-compulsive disorder	4.5
11	Insomnia (primary)	3.6	Obsessive-compulsive disorder	0.6	Post-traumatic stress disorder	3.0
12	Post-traumatic stress disorder	3.5	Epilepsy	0.5	Insomnia (primary)	2.9
13	Parkinson's disease	1.7	Post-traumatic stress disorder	0.5	Multiple sclerosis	1.2
14	Multiple sclerosis	1.5	Multiple sclerosis	0.3	Parkinson's disease	1.0

Source: adapted from reference 2.

Notes
1 WorldBank criteria for income (2009 gross national income (GNI) per capita): low income is US$995 equivalent or less; middle income is $996–12,195; high income is $12,196 or more.
2 A disability adjusted life year (DALY) is a unit measuring the amount of health lost because of a disease or injury. It is calculated as the present value of the future years of disability-free life that are lost as a result of the premature deaths or disability occurring in a particular year.

Service delivery improvement using capacity building approach

Mental health service delivery using a capacity building approach needs to address four critical areas; (1) human resources, (2) consumer participation and stigma reduction, (3) improved funding, (4) development of evidence base of effectiveness of mental health services.

Human resources

Capacity building for adequate mental health human resources entails creating regional training and research centres for mental health research, education training and practice that incorporates the views and needs of local people, sustainable models to train and increase the number of culturally and ethnically diverse mental health service providers, and strengthening the mental health component in the training of all health care personnel. The current inadequacy of skilled mental health service in providers in poor nations is illustrated in part in Figure 18.2.

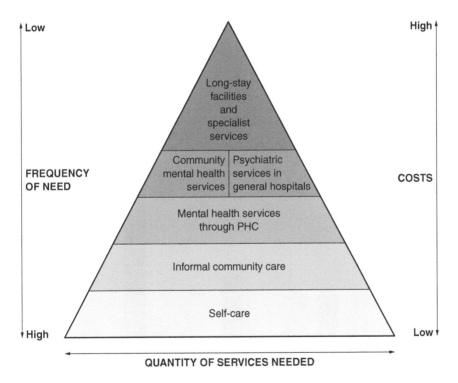

Figure 18.1 The WHO's optimal mix of mental health services (adapted from reference 5).

Apart from quantity, there is also a need to address mental health equity and distribution constraints in most nations through targeted policies and practical incentive–disincentive policies.[6]

Consumer participation and stigma reduction

Consumer participation and stigma reduction are complementary services – the more community members actively participate in the management of mental health services, the less likely that mentally ill individuals will be stigmatised. Many societies view mental illness as largely incurable and a threat to social control, and may use stigmatising practices and policies (e.g. stereotyping and discrimination) to exclude those affected by mental illness. The stigma attached to mental illness is a major obstacle to the provision of care for people with this disorder. Stigma does not stop at illness: it undesirably brands those who are ill, their families across generations, institutions that provide treatment, psychotropic drugs and mental health workers.[7] Australia's mental health policies exemplify increased commitment to consumer participation in mental health services over the past two decades.[8]

Improved funding

Although mental health and neuropsychiatric disorders constitute about 13 per cent of global burden of disease, in no nation is mental health-specific funding currently above 9 per cent of total health budget – a level

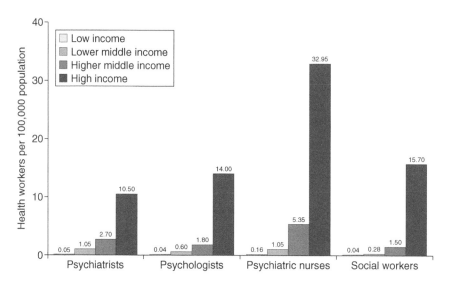

Figure 18.2 Global distribution of core mental health workers by income level (adapted from reference 9).

considered by the author as the optimal funding proportion. Australia continues to record improvements in mental health funding, both in absolute terms as well as in relation to total health expenditure.

Evidence-based mental health services

Research is important to determine a solid evidence basis for the efficiency and effectiveness of mental health services. The grand challenge in global mental health initiative recently identified 25 research priorities to improve delivery of services to people with mental and neuropsychiatric disorders.[10] Highlights include: 'Integrate screening and core packages of services into routine primary health care'; 'reduce the cost and improve the supply of effective medications'; 'provide effective and affordable community-based care and rehabilitation'; improve children's access to evidence based care in low and middle income countries'; strengthen mental health component of training of all healthcare personnel'. Capacity building for evidence-based mental health service delivery should include the development of key performance indicators (e.g. Effect Size and Reliable Change Index) such as those developed in 2008 by the Australian Health Outcomes and Classification Framework.[11]

References

1 Riese, W. The Legacy of Philippe Pinel: An Inquiry into Thought on Mental Alienation. New York: Springer Publishing Co Inc., 1969.
2 World Health Organization. Mental Health and Development: Targeting People with Mental Health Conditions as a Vulnerable Group. Geneva: WHO, 2010.
3 McGrath, J., Saha, S., Chant, D., Welham, J. Schizophrenia: a concise overview of incidence, prevalence, and mortality. *Epidemiologic Reviews*, 2008; 30: 67–76.
4 Foti, D.J., Kotov, R., Guey, L.T., Bronnet, E.J. Cannabis use and the course of schizophrenia: 10-year follow-up after first hospitalization. *American Journal of Psychiatry*, 2010; 167: 987–993.
5 World Health Organization. WHO Mental Health Services Pyramid: Mental Health Policy and Services Development. Geneva: WHO, 2003.
6 Saxena, S., Thornicroft, G., Knapp, M., Whiteford, H. Resources for mental health: scarcity, inequity, and inefficiency. *Lancet*, 2007; 370: 878–889.
7 Sartorius, N. Stigma and mental health. *Lancet*, 2007; 370: 810–811
8 Commonwealth of Australia. *National Mental Health Report, 2010*. Canberra: Australian Government, 2010.
9 World Health Organization. Human Resources for Mental Health: Workforce Shortages in Low and Middle Income Countries. Geneva: WHO, 2011.
10 Collins, P.Y., Patel, V., Joestl, S.S., March, D., Insel, T.R., Daar, A.S., *et al.* Grand challenges in global mental health. *Nature*, 2011; 475: 27–30.
11 Australian Health Outcomes and Classification Framework. Key Performance Indicators for Australian Public Mental Health Services: Developing Effectiveness KPIs from the NOCC Data. Parramatta: NSW Institute of Psychiatry, 2008.

Part V

Addressing obstacles, and evaluating capacity building activities in the health systems

19 Challenges encountered in health systems' capacity building

Health system performance

Health system performance in developing nations remain chronically inadequate and in need of urgent reforms. In the WHO 2000 World Health Report, developing nations like Myanmar and Nigeria are at the bottom of the global health systems performance rankings. Poorly developed health systems consistently fail to deliver services effectively, especially to the most vulnerable citizens. The best strategies to improve health system performance are often incremental and encompass action at all levels to address system constraints. Funding for health systems strengthening accounts for less than 0.5 per cent of the annual health expenditure of developing countries, and this level of funding should be significantly increased. The World Health Organization's health systems framework comprises building blocks and suggested outcomes (Chapter 2, Figure 2.7). Common interventions to improve health systems at each of the building blocks are shown in Table 19.1.

The following case study on the Tanzania Essential Health Interventions Project (TEHIP) illustrates the impact of health systems strengthening on health system improvement. Tanzania is an East African country whose implementation of a series of essential interventions on its health system commenced in 1996, brought about evidence-based health planning and practice in two districts, Rufiji and Morogoro. The idea is directly related to the Word Bank's *World Development Report 1993: Investing in Health,* which focused on health systems, suggesting that health could be significantly improved by adopting a minimum package of health interventions to respond directly and cost-effectively to evidence about the burden of disease. TEHIP has brought about a change in the way that local health policy and practice is planned and resources are allocated across geographical and technical areas. At the district level health care workers and managers are more in control of resources and processes. This has also contributed towards a more robust decentralisation of the health care provision.

In both districts, the introduction of TEHIP tools significantly improved budget allocation. Before TEHIP, STDs received a negligible share of total

Table 19.1 Interventions to improve health system functioning

Building block	Common types of intervention
Governance	• Decentralisation • Civil society participation • Licensure, accreditation, registration
Financing	• User fees • Conditional cash transfers (demand side) • Pay-for-performance (supply side) • Health insurance • Provider financing modalities • Sector Wide Approaches (SWAps) and basket funding
Human resources	• Integrated training • Quality improvement, performance management • Incentives for retention or remote area deployment
Information	• Shifting to electronic (versus manual) medical records • Integrated data systems and enterprise architecture for HIS design • Coordination of national household surveys (e.g. timing of data collected)
Medical products, vaccines and technologies	• New approaches to pharmacovigilance • Supply chain management • Integrated delivery of products and interventions
Service delivery	• Approaches to ensure continuity of care • Integration of services versus centrally managed programmes • Community outreach versus fixed clinics
Multiple building blocks	• Health sector reforms • District health system strengthening

Source: adapted from reference 1.

health spending (about 3 per cent). However, evidence about the burden of STDs provided by the demographic surveillance system (DSS) to health planners resulted in the increase of the share to about 9.5 per cent. Large proportional increases were also seen for malaria interventions and Integrated Management of Childhood Illnesses. These changes were made possible by new tools and a judicious use of new incremental funding from a sector-wide decentralised basket fund (on average less than US$1 per capita extra funding). Absolute per capita funds for other essential health interventions which were previously adequately funded such as immunisation, remained at their previous level. The country's health reform was receptive to decentralised, evidence-based planning and needed to find ways in which it could be implemented. Hence the opportunity to join TEHIP was welcomed at the policy level. The Tanzanian health situation and health system structure also provided an attractive context for the work of TEHIP.

The tools used to plan health evidence-based interventions included: (a) district burden of disease profile tool to repackage population health information from the DSS in a way that the district officials can easily understand; (b) district health accounts tool to analyse budgets in a standard way to generate easy-to-use graphics that show how plans for spending coalesce as a complete plan; (c) district health service mapping tool to allow health administrators to access a quick visual representation of the availability of specific health services or the attendance at health facilities for various interventions across the district; (d) community voice tools to promote community participation and inform health planning, and to promote ownership. An underlying principle and result of these health system interventions was that there was a need for integrated solutions to the problem focusing on the needs and guidance of community-level health workers and managers. TEHIP, therefore, had to develop a structure that provided a fertile ground for innovations that could be integrated into the routine of the community health case workers and managers; thus making research an intrinsic part of its work.

The impact of these interventions can now be observed. Child mortality in the two districts fell by over 40 per cent in the five years following the introduction of evidence-based planning; and death rates for men and women between 15 and 60 years old declined by 18 per cent. During the same period, the health indicators for other districts in Tanzania, and in fact across Africa, have become stagnant. This suggests that the project provided the Tanzanian health reform with the appropriate tools needed for development of an evidence-based health system and policies. The key lesson from this experience is that the burden of disease can be significantly lowered through relatively low cost investments in strengthening health systems by providing incremental, decentralised, sector-wide health basket funding and a tool kit of practical management, planning and priority-setting tools that assist an evidence-based approach. Other lessons regarding research-policy issues are: funding research and development simultaneously, and encouraging researchers and development specialists to be aware of and involved in each other's specific areas of concern, produces multiple benefits; development plans can benefit from the continuous input from researchers; links to concrete development agendas afford researchers greater credibility; funding and implementation priorities must be increasingly based upon locally owned, evidence-based plans that aim to develop the health system, maximise health and reduce inequities – this involves having exit strategies in place and health observatories to facilitate the involvement of local actors; demographic surveillance can inform policy and planning, monitor progress and also provide accountability for government and donor spending priorities and patterns.[2]

Key challenges in capacity building of health systems

The most comprehensive study of capacity building approaches for health systems as at 2010 was conducted by Management Sciences for Health's AIDSTAR-II project. Following a review of about 300 tools, programmes and approaches, this project identified four key challenges in capacity building:[3]

1   developing standardised indicators and evaluation of capacity building;
2   improving understanding of the definition and scope of capacity building;
3   enhancing local ownership of capacity building initiatives;
4   facilitating improved uptake of tools and programmes shown to improve capacity building efforts.

These challenges should raise the questions, listed in Figure 19.1, by providers of capacity building services.

The AIDSTAR-II review made the following recommendations to enhance the application in capacity building in improving health organisations.

• Capacity building must be subject to vigorous evaluations and monitoring, including the use of common definition, standards and indicators. AIDSTAR-II's two definitions of capacity building are: (a) 'any action that improves the effectiveness of individuals, organisations, networks or systems – including organisational and financial stability, programme service delivery, programme quality and growth'; (b) 'a long term process that improves the ability of an individual, group, organisation, or ecosystem to create positive change and perform better to improve public health results'.[4]

1. Have we budgeted sufficient time, money and human resources to do a thorough, participatory assessment that allows our clients to identify their strengths and weaknesses and to develop a plan of improvement?

2. Are our tools and approaches grounded in valid, tested theories (e.g. organisational, managerial, learning)?

3. Have we clearly negotiated all roles and responsibilities for the entire capacity building intervention for the donor, our client and us?

4. Are we willing to open ourselves up as an example of constant striving to make our work and our organisation more effective?

5. Does the local organisation offer the opportunity for staff to apply the new skills they've learned, and does it support them with appropriate organisational resources, systems and structures?

6. How will we monitor, evaluate and report in such a way that the results are useful to the local organisation and can be replicated and disseminated?

Figure 19.1 Important questions to guide capacity building efforts (source: reference 3).

- Capacity building must be participatory, needs based, with a focus on sustainability.
- Capacity building tools and approaches must be available and adaptable.
- Capacity building must be recognised as an essential technical discipline.

Training of capacity building staff is important. The World Bank's 'Flagship programme on Health Sector Reform and Sustainable Financing' exemplifies such training-focussed capacity building initiatives. The programme operates via both face-to-face as well as open and distance learning mode and, between 1997 and 2008, it was delivered to more than 19,400 participants in 51 nations.[5]

Given the wide extent of the health system, there can be no single capacity building provider. Stakeholders and foreign donors can contribute optimally in cash and kind to capacity building aspects for which they have the most interest. For example, the US Centers for Disease Control and Prevention (CDC) accords laboratory services high priority, and has developed a capacity building programme for this aspect of health systems. CDC assists resource-poor nations to build sustainable and integrated laboratory networks as a critical and core component of the overall health system. CDC works with the WHO and other national and international partners to assist multiple countries in Africa, Asia and Latin America to develop 'National Strategic Plans' to strengthen public health laboratory networks. Key components addressed in these plans include training and personnel retention, logistics and commodities management, facility and equipment maintenance and quality management systems across disease-wide laboratories, laboratory information systems, laboratory policies and regulatory issues.

Since 2007, CDC collaborated with the WHO and health experts from 12 African countries to launch the first ever accreditation programme for quality improvement of the continent's medical laboratories. These plans will reduce parallel disease-specific laboratory systems, building efficiency and augmenting the ability of countries to respond effectively to numerous diseases, including HIV, TB, malaria, opportunistic infections and Avian influenza. A notable accomplishment from CDC's capacity building programmes for laboratory services is the African Centre for Integrated Laboratory Training (ACILT).[6]

ACILT's Vision is to facilitate improved health standards in Africa through quality laboratory practices to combat major infectious diseases. Its Mission is to develop and present hands-on training courses for front-line laboratory staff. It also presents courses for programme managers, strategic planners and policy makers so that critical laboratory issues are understood and appropriately supported by host governments. The International Laboratory Branch of CDC's Division of Global AIDS provides ongoing technical assistance and expert instructors to ACILT for the course development and delivery. This includes working with international partners to ensure the use of standardised laboratory supplies for the courses. ACILT is responding to Africa's rapidly growing demand for a well-trained, competent and motivated laboratory workforce. It launched the first courses in the autumn of 2008 on Early Infant Diagnosis of HIV using molecular detection from dried blood spots; followed by a course on Laboratory Methods for culture and identification of Mycobacterium tuberculosis. Since then, based on the needs generated in countries, state-of-the-art courses, including Basic Medical Technician, Strengthening Laboratory Management Towards Accreditation (SLMTA), TB Smear Microscopy, Practical Approaches to Monitor and Improve the Quality of HIV Rapid Testing, BED Incidence Testing, Biosafety and Infrastructure Development, Line Probe Assay for TB, and National Laboratory Strategic Planning (NLSP) have been offered to more than 300 participants from over 20 countries in Sub-Saharan Africa, Asia and the Caribbean regions.

References

1   World Health Organization. *Systems Thinking for Health Systems Strengthening.* Geneva: WHO, 2009.
2   Neilson, S., Smutylo, T. The TEHIP spark: planning and managing health resources at the district level, a report on TEHIP and its influence on public policy. Evaluation Unit, IDRC, 2004. Available from: http://web.idrc.ca/

uploads/user-S/10826578841TEHIP_FINAL_April_20041.doc   (accessed   7 January 2011).

3   AIDSTAR-II. Challenges encountered in capacity building. Position Paper, Arlington: Management Sciences for Health, 2011.
4   Management Sciences for Health. AIDSTAR-II consensus building meeting on capacity building. Arlington, VA, 5 November 2009.
5   Shaw, P., Samaha, H. *World Bank Institute's Flagship Program on Health Sector Reform and Sustainable Financing*. Washington, DC: World Bank, 2009.
6   Centers for Disease Control and Prevention. *African Centre for Integrated Laboratory Training*. Johannesburg: CDC, 2007.

20 Assessing the impacts of organisational capacity building in health systems

Major challenges in impact assessment of capacity building

There are major methodological problems related to assessing the effectiveness and impact of capacity building efforts in health systems. These challenges include:

a   Meeting donor needs for quantification. In trying to reassure donors that capacity building efforts are yielding positive results, there is a tendency to develop over-bureaucratised systems which attempt to measure too many indicators. It is thus important to ensure that indicators selected to measure the impact of capacity building efforts are reasonable and practical to collect.[1]

b   Being multi-dimensional and user friendly. Capacity building activities in health (e.g. poverty alleviation) tend to produce multiple effects, hence the need for multi-dimensional capacity building tools. The OECD Development Cooperation Directorate for assessing effectiveness of development aid includes the following checklist.[2]

> *Relevance*: the extent to which the aid activity is suited to the priorities and policies of the target group, recipient and donor. In evaluating the relevance of a programme or a project, it is useful to consider the following questions. To what extent are the objectives of the programme still valid? Are the activities and outputs of the programme consistent with the overall goal and the attainment of its objectives? Are the activities and outputs of the programme consistent with the intended impacts and effects?
>
> *Effectiveness*: a measure of the extent to which an aid activity attains its objectives. In evaluating the effectiveness of a programme or a project, it is useful to consider the following questions. To what extent were the objectives achieved/are likely to be achieved? What were the major factors influencing the achievement or non-achievement of the objectives?

Efficiency: measures the outputs – qualitative and quantitative – in relation to the inputs. It is an economic term which signifies that the aid uses the least costly resources possible in order to achieve the desired results. This generally requires comparing alternative approaches to achieving the same outputs, to see whether the most efficient process has been adopted. When evaluating the efficiency of a programme or a project, it is useful to consider the following questions. Were activities cost efficient? Were objectives achieved on time? Was the programme or project implemented in the most efficient way compared to alternatives?

Impact: the positive and negative changes produced by a development intervention, directly or indirectly, intended or unintended. This involves the main impacts and effects resulting from the activity on the local social, economic, environmental and other development indicators. The examination should be concerned with both intended and unintended results and must also include the positive and negative impact of external factors, such as changes in terms of trade and financial conditions. When evaluating the impact of a programme or a project, it is useful to consider the following questions. What has happened as a result of the programme or project? What real difference has the activity made to the beneficiaries? How many people have been affected?

Sustainability: is concerned with measuring whether the benefits of an activity are likely to continue after donor funding has been withdrawn. Projects need to be environmentally as well as financially sustainable. When evaluating the sustainability of a programme or a project, it is useful to consider the following questions. To what extent did the benefits of a programme or project continue after donor funding ceased? What were the major factors which influenced the achievement or non-achievement of sustainability of the programme or project?

c   Demonstrating attribution is a major problem with capacity building initiatives, given its diffuse implementation approaches and the multiplicity of processes that result in specific outcomes. However, viewed from the definitional perspective of 'ability to undertake specific objectives', 'before and after' assessments may facilitate adequate attribution of capacity building measures. The MEASURE Evaluation Project is actively involved with measuring and attributing capacity building initiatives. The MEASURE capacity building indicators are shown in Table 20.1.

d   Measuring intangible changes. Particularly in health systems, 'not everything that counts can be counted', as Einstein aptly reminds us. Improved subjective well-being is an example of a capacity building outcome that, though difficult to measure, is very important from the

Table 20.1 MEASURE capacity building indicators at various levels of health systems

Capacity building level	Inputs	Process	Outputs	Intermediates outcomes
Health system	• Population per doctor • Ratio of health care spending on primary versus tertiary care • Percentage of health budget funded by external sources	• Donor coordination committee meets every six months • Collaborative 'arrangements' exist between social sectors – e.g. meetings between health and agriculture or health and education	• Number of multi-sectoral meetings held • Number of collaborative projects initiated outside health • Existence of national standards for professional qualifications • Existence of sector-wide strategy	• Widely distributed sector-wide strategy • Regular auditing of system-wide accounts by independent company
Organisation	• Existence of clear mission statement • Presence of operational planning system • Presence of detailed job descriptions • Clearly defined organisational structure	• Coordination with other organisations evident through internal reporting mechanisms • Job descriptions are regularly updated to reflect real work requirements and responsibilities	• Presence of a financial management system that regularly provides income/revenue data and cash flow analysis • Capacity to track commodities • Individual work plans are prepared for all staff • A sufficient number of sites functioning as clinical training sites to meet clinic practice needs	• Realised operational targets • Ability to adjust services in response to evaluation results or emergencies • Reports generated on time • Cost-sharing revenue as a proportion of the annual MOH non-wage recurrent budget • Percentage of trained health workers that correctly diagnose 2–4 months after training

Health personnel	• Adequacy of the training material/supplies has been assessed in 1 or more institutions • Adequate training supplies available in sufficient quantities to support ongoing RH/FP training in 1/more institutions	• Number of training sessions to improve human resource capacity which focus on needs identified by the service providing institution • Percentage of courses where training methodology is appropriate for transfer of skills/knowledge	• Number of providers trained, by type of training and cadre of provider • Number of staff trained in finance, MIS, strategic planning, financial planning • Number of managers trained, by type of training	• Percentage of trainees (providers) competent in skill (i.e. met set standard when applying skill learned in training) • Percentage of trainees who apply skills (learned through training) to their subsequent work
Individual/ community	• Average level of education (number of years) attained in the district • Mean income level • Proportion whose partner recently died in central hospital • Existence of community leadership	• Percentage who think they are at risk of contracting serious illness • Percentage who report previous poor experience of the health care system • Level of community cohesiveness	• Proportion of non-users who desire to use contraception in the future • Level of participation in community health committees	• Percentage of new mothers who bring their children for immunisation at the right time • Proportion of individuals who adhere to appropriate/given drug regime • Level of community mobilisation and empowerment

Source: adapted from reference 3.

perspective of health consumers. Many measures of institutional and organisational capacity are subjective, and rely mainly on individual judgment and perception, thus limiting their reliability and generalisability. Harmony in working relationships between the various components of health systems is vital for efficient functioning, but it is difficult to measure or attribute to capacity building efforts.

e   Ensuring adequacy of skills to conduct impact assessment is a major challenge in capacity building efforts, in part due to low priority accorded such activities during health sector budgeting processes. Self-assessment may create conflict of interest issues, which might result in data manipulation in order to present results in favourable light. On the other hand, internal stakeholders may mistrust external evaluators, and misconstrue evaluation tools as a ploy for sanctions. This potential challenge may be addressed through prior agreement of the personnel and tools that will be utilised in the conduct of impact assessment.

f   Overall cost-effectiveness of impact assessment processes. Meaningful capacity building assessment is expensive, and its utility is strongly conditioned by assessment tools, organisational knowledge and level of investment in the evaluation process. Two approaches to determining evaluation budgets are to limit the total amount authorised, or to link it to the total budget (e.g. maximum 0.5 per cent of total budget). Evaluation personnel are best selected from a wide section of stakeholders.

Credible capacity building impact assessment approaches

Addressing capacity building impact assessment challenges entails paying particular attention to the issues summarised in Table 20.2. There are scores of capacity building assessment tools in current use, which are appropriate at organisational and health system levels. For example, the WHO-supported Gender, Women and Health Network (GWHN) developed a tool for assessing policy coherence in human rights and policy coherence in health sector strategies. The tool was designed to support countries to strengthen national health strategies by applying human rights and gender equality commitments and obligations. The tool poses critical questions to identify gaps and opportunities in the review or reform of health sector strategies. Evaluation of its feasibility in a national assessment of human rights and gender equality in Yemen were largely positive.[4]

In utilising instruments to evaluate the impact of capacity building in health organisations and health systems, it is important to first determine whether the assessment is motivated from within or outside an organisation. Evaluators need to determine four points: (1) the central purpose of the assessment; (2) the time and budget; (3) the overall approach; (4) how to communicate and use the information. These matters are

Table 20.2 Capacity building assessment variables

Strategy	Measurement issue addressed
Utilise participatory processes as intervention	Multiple understanding of terms Evolving understanding of capacity Building trust and dealing with sensitive issue
Acknowledge the context	Invisibility of capacity building Dynamic context
Incorporate mixed methods (qualitative and quantitative)	Invisibility of capacity building Dynamic context Time course for change Building trust and dealing with sensitive issues 'Snap-shot' measures Validity and reliability of quantitative methods Attribution for change in capacity
Build on previous phases of community and stakeholder engagement	Multiple understanding of terms Building trust and dealing with sensitive issues
Establish validity of quantitative measures	Validity and reliability of quantitative methods
Establish trustworthiness of qualitative intelligence	Multiple understanding of terms Evolving understanding of capacity Time course for change Building trust and dealing with sensitive issues 'snap-shot' measures
Be flexible and adaptive	Dynamic context Multiple understanding of terms Building trust and dealing with sensitive issues
Identify intervention contribution, i.e. intervention specific evaluations	Attribution for change in capacity

ideally contained in written terms of reference that help clarify and communicate the intentions. The form of those terms will vary for an external assessment versus a self-assessment, but, in either case, they are useful in keeping the process and vision of the assessment's objectives on track. Many assessments suffer from poorly prepared terms of reference that are little more than a compilation of questions from various stakeholders. Such terms of reference reflect inexperience and need to be re-cast before a productive assessment can begin. This can be accomplished by better conceptualising the work plan that responds to the terms of reference.[5]

The international capacity building agency known as Management Sciences for Health recently developed a tool for assessing capacity building efforts in fragile health systems. The tool comprises six critical management areas; oversight and coordination, human resources, resource management, health financing, community involvement and health information management. The questionnaire-based tool was recently trialled in four counties in the poor African nation of Liberia, with promising outcomes in relation to reliability and validity (Table 20.3).

The findings reflect a sub-optimal management of health systems in the reviewed nationally representative counties of Liberia. Such findings set the stage for structured capacity development programmes for health system management. Based on their findings, the authors proposed the following recommendations for improving Liberia's health system:[6]

- define county health teams' roles in health services management and integrate health planning at central and county levels;
- address severe inadequacies in quality, quantity and distribution of health staff, in part by expanding public health services continuing health professionals' education and open–distance learning;

Table 20.3 Summary of Liberia's health management capacity, by county and system components

Health system component	Bomi County	Bong County	Gran Cape Mount County	Nimba County	Average
1 Oversight and coordination	2	2	2	2	2
2 Human resources	2	2	2	2	2
3 Resource management	1	1	1	1	1
4 Health financing	1	3	1	1	1.5
5 Community participation	1	1	3	1	1.5
6 Information management	2	2	2	2	2
Average county score	1.5	1.8	1.8	1.5	–

Source: adapted from reference 6.

Notes
Key: 1, minimal or no management capacity evident; 2, some basic management capacity present, but quite marginal; 3, strong management capacity present.

- develop human and financial resources' management capacity;
- establish and expand health management information systems to strengthen the use of health information.

A major reason for the tool's success is community ownership, with local surveyors and health ministry officials playing prominent roles in the assessment process.[5]

References

1   Hailey, J., James, R. NGO capacity building: the challenge of impact assessment. Paper presented to the 'New Directions in Impact Assessment for Development Methods and Practice' conference, Manchester, 2003.

2   Organization for Economic Cooperation and Development (OECD). *Glossary of Terms Used in Evaluation, in 'Methods and Procedures in Aid Evaluation'*. Brussels: OECD, 1986.

3   Brown, L., LaFond, A., MacIntyre, K. *Measuring Capacity Building.* Chapel Hill, NC, MEASURE Evaluation, Carolina Population Center, 2001.

4   World Health Organization. *Human Rights and Gender Equality in Health Sector Strategies: How to Assess Policy Coherence.* Geneva: WHO, 2011.

5   Lusthaus, C., Adrian, M.H., Anderson, G., Carden, F., Mantalvian, P. *Organizational Assessment: A Framework for Improving Performance.* Washington, DC: Inter-American Development Bank, and International Development Research Centre, Canada, 2002.

6   Newbrander, W., Peercy, C., Shepherd-Banigan, M., Vergeer, P. A tool for assessing management capacity at the decentralised level in a fragile state. *International Journal of Health Planning and Management,* 2011; DOI: 10.1002/hpm.1108.

Epilogue

Capacity is one of the core determinants of organisational performance. A need for capacity building is often identified when performance is inadequate. Capacity building interventions work to improve the processes that occur within the entire health system, including the organisation of the health system, health personnel and health consumers. Organisational capacity building in health is characterised by being a multi-dimensional, dynamic process; measurable at four levels of society: health system, organisation, health personnel and individual/community; effective implementation should result in improvements in health performance and outcomes at each of these levels; it contributes to the sustainability of health systems; it is influenced by the external environment.[2] Important capacity building domains are summarised in Table E.1.

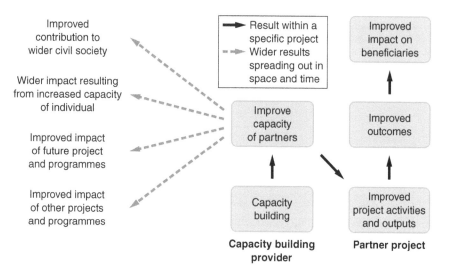

Figure E.1 Illustration of changes that occur as a result of improved capacity building (adapted from reference 1).

Table E.1 Capacity building domains

Domain	Description
Participation	Participation is basic to community empowerment. Only by participating in small groups or larger organisations can individual community members better define, analyse and act on issues of general concern to the broader community.
Leadership	Participation and leadership are closely connected. Leadership requires a strong participant base just as participation requires the direction and structure of strong leadership. Both play an important role in the development of small groups and community organisations.
Organisational structures	Organisational structures in a community include small groups such as committees, and church and youth groups. These are the organisational elements which represent the ways in which people come together in order to socialise, and to address their concerns and problems. The existence of and the level at which these organisations function is crucial to community empowerment.
Problem assessment	Empowerment presumes that the identification of problems, solutions to the problems and actions to resolve the problems are carried out by the community. The process assists communities to develop a sense of self-determination and capacity.
Resource mobilisation	The ability of the community both to mobilise resources from within and to negotiate resources from beyond the community is an important factor in its ability to achieve successes in its efforts.
'Asking why'	The ability of the community to critically assess the social, political, economic and other causes of inequality is a crucial stage towards developing appropriate personal and social change strategies.
Links with others	Links with people and organisations, including partnerships, coalitions and voluntary alliances between the community and others, can assist the community in addressing its issues.
Role of the outside agents	In a programme context, outside agents are often an important link between communities and external resources. Their role is especially important near the beginning of a new programme, when the process of building new community momentum may be triggered and nurtured. The outside agent increasingly transforms power relationships between her/himself, outside agencies and the community, such that the community assumes increasing programme authority.
Programme management	Programme management that empowers the community includes the control by the primary stakeholders over decisions on planning, implementation, evaluation, finances, administration, reporting and conflict resolution. The first step towards programme management by the community is to clearly define the roles, responsibilities and line management of all stakeholders.

Source: adapted from reference 2.

Organisational capacity building efforts in health systems exemplify the ripple effect in the sense that when properly and sustainably implemented, their effects go beyond those related to the specified project to those spreading out in space and time (Figure E.1). Within the specified project, the impact is felt at all levels (Figure E.2).

Organisational and health systems capacity building approaches significantly influence the perspectives of health managers and leaders in relation to addressing health problems. The tools required for a disease specific response are not always identical to those required for a health system response (Table E.2).

A capacity building approach facilitates the choice of appropriate tools and their expert application. Although disease-focussed responses may be implemented relatively quickly and are generally less difficult to monitor and evaluate, multiple disease-specific programmes are unsustainable and create major coordination problems for health managers and front-line staff.

Given its potential positive roles in health organisation and health system improvement, it is surprising that very few public health schools teach capacity building as part of the health curriculum. When public health workers, civil society organisations and health policy makers hold capacity building to the highest standards, it will maintain health programmes and structures at the high levels of quality and effectiveness. Organisational and systems capacity building is critical to the development of health systems, and should be accorded high priority in health

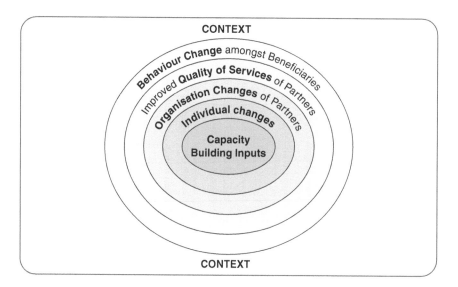

Figure E.2 The ripple model in relation to organisational capacity building in health systems (adapted from reference 3).

Table E.2 Disease specific and health system responses to selected health constraints

Constraint	Disease-specific response	Health system response
Financial inaccessibility, inability to pay, informal fees	Allowing exemptions or reducing prices for focal diseases	Developing risk-pooling strategies
Physical inaccessibility: distance to facility	Providing outreach for focal diseases	Reconsidering long-term plans for capital investment and siting of facilities
Inappropriately skilled staff	Organising in-service training workshops to develop skills in focal diseases	Reviewing basic medical and nursing curricula to ensure that basic training includes appropriate skills
Poorly motivated staff	Offering financial incentives for the delivery of particular priority services	Instituting performance review systems, creating greater clarity about roles and expectations, reviewing salary structures and promotion procedures
Weak planning and management	Providing ongoing education and training workshops to develop planning and management skills	Restructuring ministries of health, recruiting and developing a cadre of dedicated managers
Lack of intersectional action and partnership	Creating disease-focused, cross-sectorial committees and task forces at the national level	Building systems of local government that incorporate representatives from health, education and agriculture, promoting the accountability of local governance structures to the people
Poor quality care among private sector providers	Offering training for private sector providers	Developing accreditation and regulation systems

Source: adapted from reference 4.

professionals' education and health projects' management. Capacity building offers significant opportunities for innovations – defined as practices which facilitate sustainability of health systems and health improvements through executing 'game-changing' ideas – within health systems.

The health promotion era of public health was instrumental in making capacity building programmes central to organisational and health systems development practice. With the ascendancy of the population health era of public health, it is important to elevate the status of capacity building as a major tool in public health and organisational improvement strategies. This book is a modest contribution towards reviving the capacity building concept in health organisations and health systems.

References

1   Simister, N., Smith, R. Monitoring and evaluating capacity building: is it really that difficult? Praxis Paper 23. International NGO Research and Training Centre, 2010.
2   Brown, L., LaFond, A., MacIntyre, K. Measuring capacity building. Chapel Hill, NC, MEASURE Evaluation, Carolina Population Center, 2001.
3   Hailey, J., James, R. NGO capacity building: the challenge of impact assessment. Conference presentation, IDPM: University of Manchester, 2003. Available from http://portals.wi.wur.nl/files/docs/ppme/Hailey.pdf (accessed 2 April 2012).
4   Travis, P., Bennett, S., Hains, A., Pang, T., Bhutta, Z., Hyder, A.A., *et al.* Overcoming health system constraints to achieve the Millennium Development Goals. *Lancet*; 2004; 364: 900–906.

Index

Page numbers in *italics* denote tables, those in **bold** denote figures.